THE WORLD'S BEST
MASSAGE
TECHNIQUES

THE COMPLETE ILLUSTRATED GUIDE

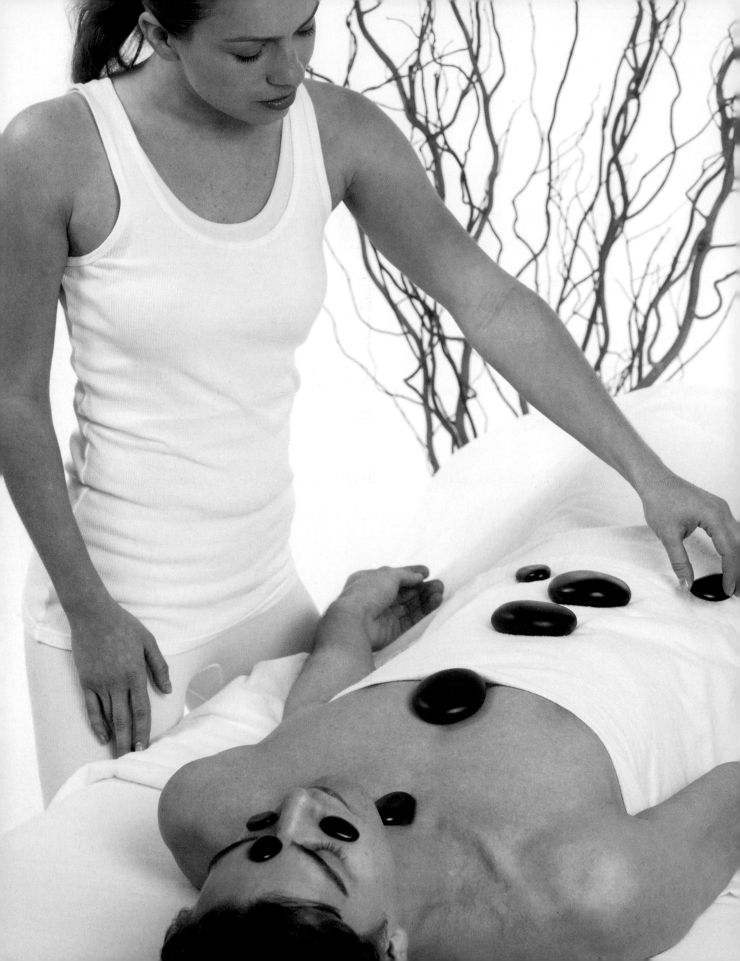

THE WORLD'S BEST

MASSAGE TECHNIQUES

THE COMPLETE ILLUSTRATED GUIDE

INNOVATIVE BODYWORK
PRACTICES FROM AROUND
THE GLOBE FOR PLEASURE,
RELAXATION, AND PAIN RELIEF

VICTORIA JORDAN STONE, N.C.M.T.

First published in the USA in 2010 by
Fair Winds Press, a member of
Quayside Publishing Group
100 Cummings Center
Suite 406-L
Beverly, MA 01915-6101
www.fairwindspress.com

14 13 12 11 10   1 2 3 4 5

ISBN-13: 978-1-59233-430-8
ISBN-10: 1-59233-430-X

Library of Congress Cataloging-in-Publication Data available

Cover design by Kathie Alexander
Book design by Kathie Alexander
Photography by Luciana Pampalone

Printed and bound in Singapore

The information in this book is for educational purposes only. It is not intended to replace the advice of a physician or medical practitioner. Please see your health care provider before beginning any new health program.

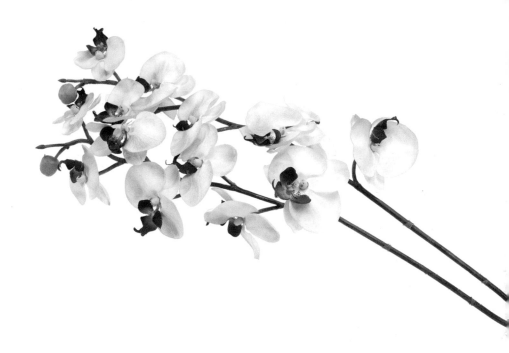

This book is dedicated to Lloyd Winfree Stone, who instilled in me the habit of lifelong learning, and to Susie Schulze, who personified the spirit of giving.

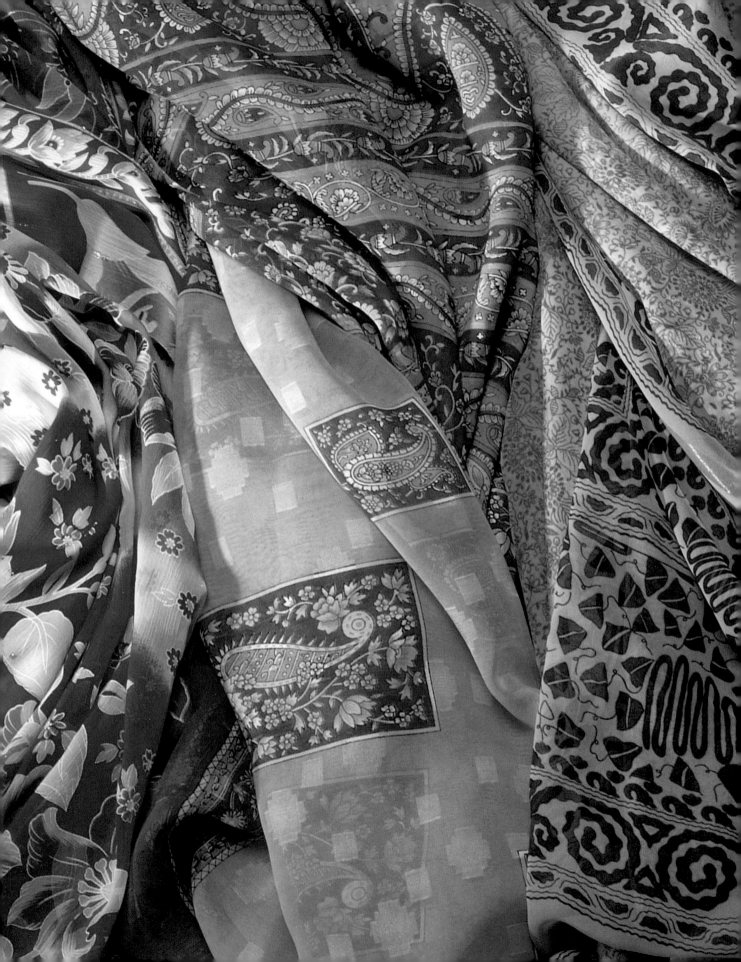

CONTENTS

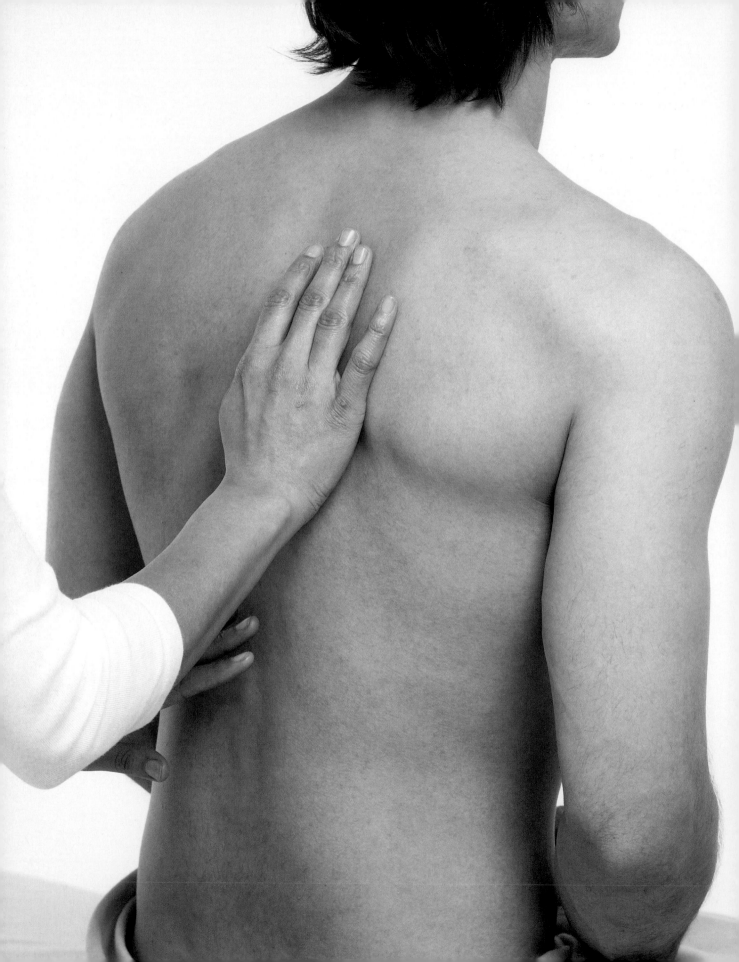

A World of Comfort in Touch

Touch is our earliest sense, primal and pleasurable. Being able to skillfully touch a person you care about is a great blessing for both of you. You can provide your child, spouse, parent, sibling, or friend with comfort, relief from discomfort, relaxation, harmony, wellness, and balance.

Are you one of those "touchy-feely" people who can't recall a time you were not massaging other people's aching necks or backs? Perhaps you'd like to try some new techniques and are curious about the differences in massage from various cultures. In this book, you will learn how to skillfully apply a wide variety of techniques from other cultures and enhance the well-being of those with whom you share massage.

We cannot touch without being touched, and this applies at all levels: physical, emotional, energetic, spiritual, and relational. One of the great blessings of massage is that the giver frequently receives as much benefit as the receiver. For that reason, we often refer in this book to the person receiving the massage as your "partner." This book is not intended as a manual for therapeutic massage, which is best left to certified and licensed individuals, nor is partner meant to indicate a level of intimate relationship.

These massage techniques are meant to be used for relaxation, stress relief, and wellness for healthy individuals. If your partner has any health problems, a physician should be consulted to provide a release for her to receive massage. The techniques are not meant to be treatments but rather to enhance the general well-being of the people you care about. If you find there are parts of one form you and your partner enjoy, there is absolutely no reason why you can't integrate those parts with another massage modality.

I highly recommend you learn the Swedish massage sequence before the others and especially before hot stone massage and lomi lomi. As you read each chapter, set up a practice area and keep the book at hand. Try a form several times before moving to the next one, so you really get a feel for each modality of massage. Four of the forms are practiced on a mat and four are table-based, but you can adapt most to mat or massage table. To understand some of the less-familiar terminology, please refer to chapter 9 before you continue with the specific forms of massage. There, you will also find useful information about setup and preparation for massage.

Although the instructions are very specific, you always may modify them according to your partner's preferences and what feels right for your own body. Massage is an art; enjoy learning and practicing in ways that will feel good for you as well as your partner. Exercise your creativity and have fun!

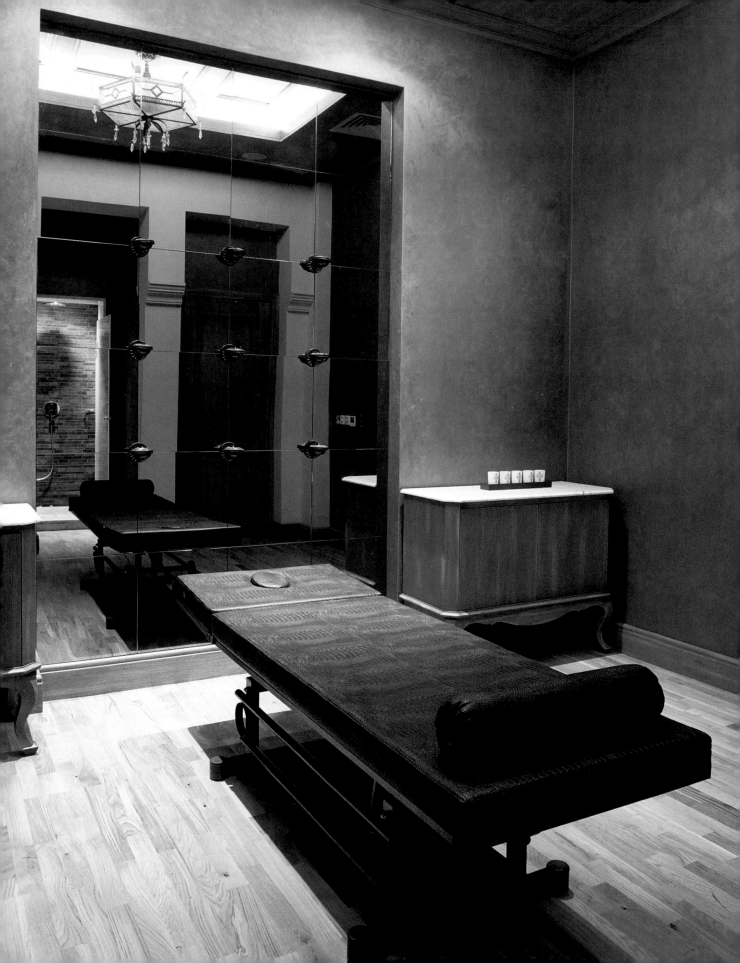

CHAPTER 1

Swedish Massage Sets the Stage

In the West, what most people think of when they hear the word massage is Swedish massage, a system directly applied to the skin that includes gliding, kneading, and percussive strokes; friction; compression; vibration; and range of motion. Lubricants such as creams, lotions, or oils are used to facilitate smooth movements of the hands over the skin of the receiver. Swedish massage is performed on a massage table, and most sessions are between thirty and ninety minutes long.

Prepare the Room and Your Body for Comfort

The room should be warm—72°F–74°F (22°C–23°C) is optimal—and with at least 3 feet (91.4 cm) of cleared area on each side of the massage table. The table height should be set where you can place the backs of your fingers from your knuckles on the table surface as you stand up straight and allow your arm to hang down loosely. If you find you are elevating your shoulders when you apply massage strokes, you should lower the height of the table; if you are bending over, bring the table height up. Have a chair or stool ready at the head of the massage table. Its height should allow you to place your forearms on the surface of the table with your shoulders in a neutral, not elevated, position.

It may be useful to perform some hand and arm stretches and do some lunges and squats to warm up your legs before you begin massage, as flexing your knees is the best way to adjust your own height relative to the table height as you are massaging.

LINENS, LUBE, AND LIGHTING

Use mostly cotton or flannel twin sheets on the massage table; your partner will lie on the fitted sheet with the flat sheet covering her body. A blanket or bath towel measuring about 4' x 6' (1.2 x 1.8 m) may be used over the sheet if your partner becomes chilled as she relaxes, which often happens. A pillow for use under her knees

Receivers Should Bathe, Not Eat, before a Session

Your partner should not have a large meal immediately prior to a massage session and may want to shower or bathe so that the lubricant, which is nutritive for the skin, may remain on her body and be fully absorbed, preferably for several hours or overnight.

Use Light Pressure and Slowly Deepen

Swedish massage begins with large, broad movements and gradually moves into smaller and more specific actions as the tissues warm up and become soft. You apply massage lightly, or superficially, at the beginning of a session, while you are spreading the lubricant and introducing yourself to your partner's body; you gradually deepen the pressure as you palpate or feel for inconsistencies and "issues" in the muscles.

When in doubt, always work with less pressure than you think is required and apply the strokes slowly. Watch for any indication that something is uncomfortable, such as facial grimaces, changes in breathing patterns, or clenched hands. Ask your partner if she is experiencing any discomfort and adjust your strokes accordingly.

Swedish massage does not work deeply into tissues, and heavy people require no more pressure than thin ones. Amateurs should not work on athletes; they are likely to injure themselves trying to work deeply, when in fact, athletes benefit more in performance and after events from superficial, repetitive work.

should be close at hand. Some people enjoy having a rice or flaxseed-filled eye pillow or neck roll, which may be microwaved to provide soothing heat. The eye pillow may also be placed in the freezer for a refreshing, cool eye compress.

Have lubricant available, warmed to room temperature. Buy small portions of various types so that you can determine which lotion you prefer. Some manufacturers of professional massage lubricants will provide you with small sample sizes at an attractively low price. Adding two or three drops of fragrant lavender, tangerine, bergamot, grapefruit, or ylang-ylang high-quality essential oil from your local health food store can provide a relaxing and refreshing quality to the massage.

Lighting should be low, not overhead. Quiet, slow music is a nice addition to the experience.

Swedish Strokes and Repetitions

Use your intuition to determine the number of stroke repetitions to use throughout the massage. Usually, at least two or three repetitions of a particular stroke are required for someone to relax into them and know what to anticipate. Repeating a stroke more than ten times will get boring at best and aggravating at worst, so somewhere between three and six reps is a good guideline.

Effleurage—Using the flat palm with fingers together, you glide away from your torso with neutral (not flexed or hyperextended) wrists. Effleurage strokes may be performed with one or both hands or with forearms in some areas of the body. While most effleurage strokes are one long flowing excursion along a body part, pushing strokes are short strokes with alternating hands; one hand chases the other along an area of the body. Pushing strokes are alternating effleurage with the palms.

Friction—Small circles or short back-and-forth movements applied with the fingers or thumbs

Stripping—Short friction strokes applied in the direction of the muscle fibers

Petrissage—Kneading, lifting, and squeezing muscle tissue with the palm in full contact with the skin

Spreading strokes—A type of effleurage stroke in which the hands move apart to stretch the skin and underlying muscles

Compression—Pressing downward into the tissue, with fingers, thumbs, or palms

Wringing—Grasping an area, usually of a limb, and working your hands in opposition to each other, as if wringing water out of a towel

Supine Upper Body Sequence: Starting with the Head and Neck Relaxes the Entire Person

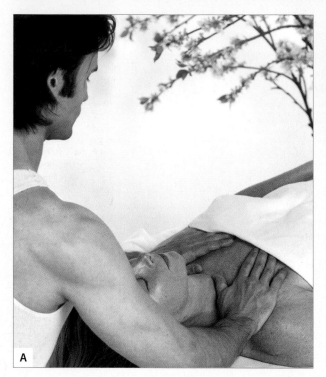

A

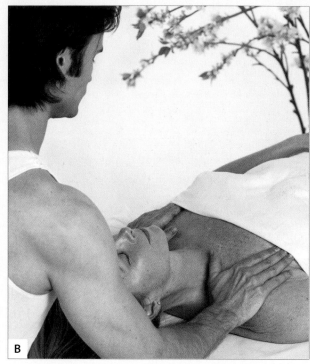

B

The goal of all Swedish massage is relaxation, stress relief, and overall well-being. This face-up sequence addresses tension in the head, face, neck, and shoulders and relieves discomfort in overworked arms, hands, and legs. Many people think of massage as starting face down, but relaxing the head and neck has the effect of relaxing the whole person, which is a productive way to begin.

1. PREPARATION AND FEEDBACK

When your partner lies on the massage table, have her lift her knees and place a pillow beneath them and her lower thighs. This will reduce strain on her lower back. Make sure she is comfortable and warm enough. Ask her to give you constructive feedback on your massage, letting you know what feels especially good and what adjustments you could make in your strokes to improve her massage experience.

Begin seated at the head of the massage table. Place your hands lightly on your partner's lateral shoulders or upper chest or cup her head without placing your hands on her ears. Your hands should be relaxed in this contact hold and stationary for about three to five breaths. This gives you an opportunity to bring your focus on her by following her breath and allows her to relax into your initial touch. Begin and end each section of her body with a contact hold.

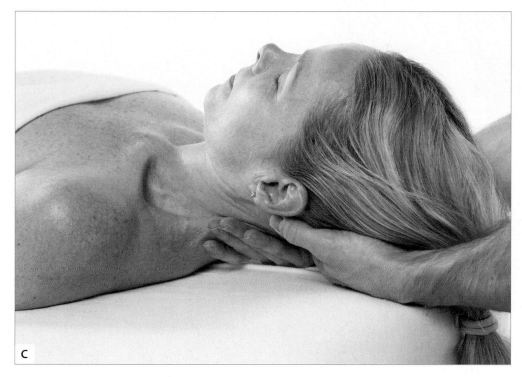

C

**Warning!
Avoid Touching the
Ear Unintentionally**

Avoid placing your hands
over your partner's ears,
banging them, or drag-
ging any part of your
hands over her ears while
you are massaging her
head and neck. It is fine
to specifically perform
delicate and intentional
massage on the ears, but
it can be intensely irritating for your partner to
receive unintentional ear
contact. Also, you should
try to avoid pushing
your partner's hair into
her ears, and instead,
try to sweep it away
from them.

Open the Chest and Lengthen the Neck

Bring your hands to the center of your partner's
upper chest and perform a spreading stroke all
the way out and around her shoulders (photos
A and B). Rotate your wrists laterally and come
under her shoulders to her neck, with your
palms up. When your hands arrive at the back
of her neck, cup the palm and fingers of one
hand around your partner's neck and glide all
the way up to the back of her head. As that
hand comes past the base of her skull, use your
other hand to cup her neck and follow your
first hand, supporting her neck fully before you
take the first hand off (photo C). Continue with
alternating hand-pulling strokes up the back of
her neck for two or three repetitions.

Your hands should graze the surface of the
massage table, keeping your partner's neck in a
neutral position as you perform this profoundly
relaxing, lengthening stroke. If your partner has
difficulty relaxing her head and neck, ask her to
allow her head to be heavy in your hands. Repeat this move from the center of the chest at
least three times. Most of us are so accustomed
to holding tension in our necks that receiving
lengthening massage strokes can help the
body remember how to relax and avoid chronically tight necks and resultant headaches.

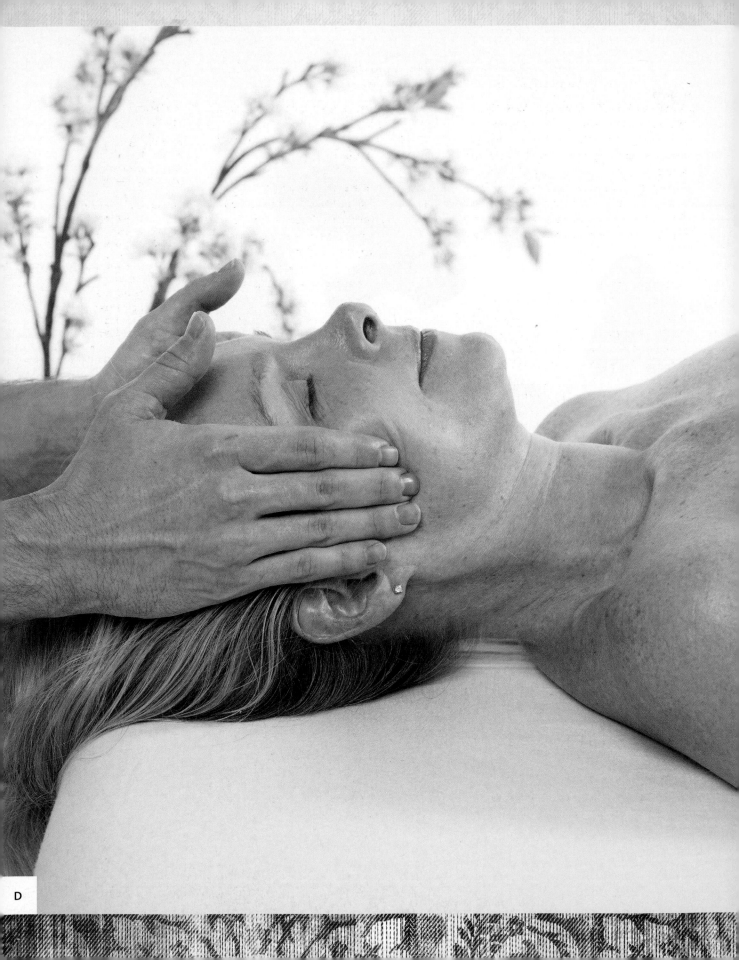

2. MASSAGE THE FACE, HEAD, AND NECK

With your palms facing down, bring your thumbs together in the middle of your partner's forehead. Linger there with light pressure for a breath; then perform a spreading stroke all the way out to where her cheek meets the front of her ear. Spreading the forehead two or three times can help alleviate the troublesome vertical lines between our eyebrows that result from squinting or frowning.

Perform a Face Lift

Bring your fingertips together under your partner's chin and sweep your hands slowly up the side of her face to the top of her head a few times, which works like a little face lift. Bring your fingers to the side of her nose and trace below her cheekbones out to the front of her ear. You will feel a small indentation right in front of her ear. This is an acupressure point you can compress gently for about thirty seconds to help relieve head pain. Two other acupressure points lie along the same path you have traced: At the nose crease and midway between the nose crease and the headache point, right below the cheekbones, are sinus points. Compressing them lightly for thirty seconds frequently will relieve nasal congestion. Make a few tracings below your partner's cheekbone laterally, pausing on the points if they feel good to her.

Soften the Jaw Muscle

The only place on the face you should perform downward strokes is on the lateral face at the jaw (**photo D**). The masseter muscle is one of the strongest muscles in the body, and if you have your partner clench her teeth briefly it is easy to find. Make several short, downward stripping strokes on this muscle to help create length and ease in it, but don't use so much pressure that you aggravate the muscle tension. Tension often lodges in this muscle, as does anger, and grinding the teeth or chewing gum can create jaw, neck, and head pain that

may be relieved by massaging this muscle. Try some circular friction strokes on the masseter as well and end with a stationary compression for a breath or two.

Circles on the Base of the Skull

Bring the backs of your wrists to the table surface so that your fingertips curve upward at the base of your partner's skull (the occipital ridge) and apply circular friction back and forth across the ridge with your hands mirroring each other. Close your eyes and really allow your fingertips to do all the "seeing" for you, feeling for taut bands and knots, and pausing to just compress them for a breath when you detect them. Continue the circular friction up and down your partner's neck on each side of her spine, still palpating for areas that are tight or knotty.

Tension stored in the neck from emotional stress, working at a computer, driving, and many other work activities may be eased by compressing the tight areas you find while you instruct your partner to visualize directing breath into tight areas, or "breathe into the area," loosening the knots and bands, which will seem to melt under your fingers. If you feel your partner tensing her neck at all, seek her feedback on how it feels and lighten your pressure while reducing the speed of your circles on her neck.

Coin Rubs around the Ear

Now for those intentional ear strokes: Take your partner's ear lobes between your thumbs and forefingers and make circles with your fingertips, gradually moving up and around the whole external ear. Then position your hands so that your partner's ears are between your index and middle fingers and make about a 1-inch (2.5 cm) stroke downward toward her jaw, easing the pressure as you slide your fingers back up; repeat this stroke several times. Your partner will enjoy this relaxing stroke as much as your dog does, but perhaps she will not drool.

You Don't Need to Be a Pro

Swedish massage is the basic form used by almost all professional massage therapists, but it is also a very accessible form for nonprofessionals to use on friends and family members for wellness and stress reduction. It has positive benefits for all the physiological systems of the body and is a wonderful form of massage for reducing discomfort, exercising creativity, and enhancing connection with another person.

Warning! Watch the Face for Grimaces

Throughout the massage, watch your partner's face for any slight grimace or indication that your pressure is not comfortable. Never hesitate to ask for feedback about how the massage is feeling. Thank your partner for sharing what she is feeling and adjust your strokes to maximize her comfort and the benefits of the massage. Never give your partner the kind of massage you want; instead, provide her with what is comfortable and useful for her.

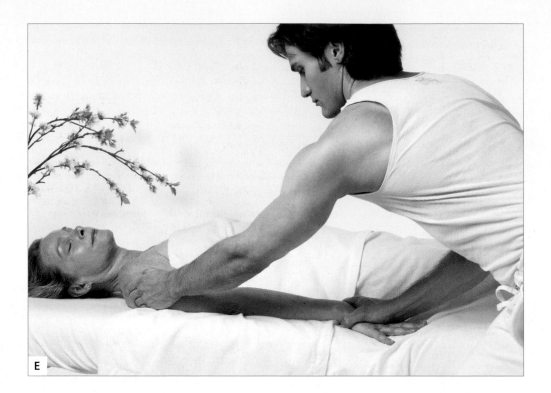

E

Pulling Strokes for the Neck

Perform several more alternating hand-pulling strokes on your partner's neck; then take her head to the left, holding it at her occiput, while your right hand glides all the way down the side of her neck and around her shoulder from front to back, then back up to her ear a few times, lengthening the muscles of the lateral neck. Repeat on the other side. Bring your partner's head back to the center and place your palms very lightly over her eyelids for a few breaths. This can be very relaxing for the eyes.

3. LUBRICATE AND LENGTHEN THE RIGHT ARM

Move to your partner's right side and spread lubricant from her fingertips up her arm and all the way around her shoulder with your left hand while you hold her right hand in your own (**photo E**). Keep enough downward tension on her arm with your right hand so that you do not force her shoulder up toward her

ear with the application of several superficial effleurage strokes with your right hand. Glide your hands much more lightly as they return from her shoulder to her hand on each stroke, as you want to encourage circulation back toward her heart.

"Milk" the Hands and Fingers

Using both your left and right hands, perform a milking stroke on your partner's hand, alternating squeezing pulls on the thumb and pinky sides of her hand for a few times each, allowing her wrist to rotate and move from side to side. This loosens the wrist and may improve flexibility and comfort in the joint, which we use constantly in almost all of our daily activities. Squeeze each finger, using a twisting motion as you move from her knuckles to her fingertips. Glide your thumbs from her knuckles to the dorsal wrist on both sides of each metacarpal bone in her hand; these bones descend from each finger through the hand.

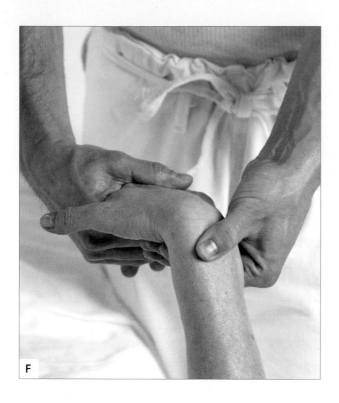

F

Strokes Return Blood to the Heart

Since Swedish massage is a circulatory type of massage, it is important to perform strokes toward the heart on the arms and legs so that blood and lymph are encouraged to return toward the heart. The intention of providing relaxation informs all the movements in Swedish massage. The variations in Swedish massage come from differing qualities of strokes, including direction, length, speed, rhythm, continuity, depth, pressure, duration, and sequence, making it possible to creatively customize a session.

Circular Friction on the Wrist

Apply circular friction on the back of your partner's wrist, increasing the pliability of the retinaculum, which is the connective tissue that encircles the wrist like a bracelet. Firmly hold your partner's wrist between your right thumb and fingers, with your thumb on the top of the joint. With your left hand, flex her wrist downward, allowing the skin and connective tissue to slide under the firm pressure of your thumb. Move your thumb medially and laterally along the back of your partner's wrist as you repeatedly flex her wrist to pull the retinaculum through, loosening it (photo F).

Maintaining malleability in the wrist can be valuable in helping to prevent carpal tunnel syndrome. You may also wring your partner's wrist; this move is like the Indian burns children give each other, but with lubricant the experience is much more pleasant.

Stretch the Palm

Allow your partner's arm to move away from the side of the table as you rotate her palm to face upward; otherwise, keeping her arm straight at her side will bind her elbow, which is uncomfortable and not the way the elbow naturally seeks to move. Apply circular friction with both of your thumbs to her palm, as you spread her palm by placing the pinkies of both of your hands between her thumb and index finger on one side of her hand and between her ring finger and pinky on the other side. This may feel awkward at first, but you just need to have your fingers between hers enough to spread her palm open. Most people are unaware of how much the small muscles in the palm are used until you begin massaging them. All of our gripping and manipulative gestures with the hands close the palm; stretching it open as you massage it will create greater flexibility and will make the whole hand feel much more open.

Knead the Forearm

Hold your partner's left hand in yours so that her wrist is almost above her elbow and use your right hand to knead the muscles in her forearm. Just as with the neck, you are likely to find lots of ropey areas and knots in the forearms because most of the muscles that give us fine-motor dexterity in our hands are located there. Allow your fingers to linger and compress any tight areas you find. Switch hands and hold her left hand in your right hand while you petrissage (lift, wring, and squeeze) the forearm muscles on the other side of her forearm with your left hand.

Fold the Arm across the Chest

Lay your partner's arm loosely across her torso and apply gentle pressure with your left hand on the back of her upper arm (photo H). Reach under her shoulder with your right hand and curl your fingers around the medial border of her scapula (shoulder blade), applying firm circular friction as you rock her upper arm away from you. You can find your partner's rhythm by rocking her arm away and experiencing how quickly it moves back to you when you release pressure but keep your hand in contact with her arm for the rocking motion. As your right hand loosens the upper back muscles between the shoulder blades, your partner's arm will gradually move closer to her chest, letting you know you have released the upper back muscles, which may be tight from general tension or from lifting activities.

Knead the Upper Arm

Lightly grasp immediately below your partner's elbow with your right hand and come to the head of the table, holding her forearm while you petrissage the back of her upper arm (the triceps muscle) with your left hand (photo G). Her elbow should be directly over her shoulder because it will feel balanced there, and she will be less likely to try to hold it up for you.

Then switch the holding hand and knead your partner's upper arm (biceps) with your

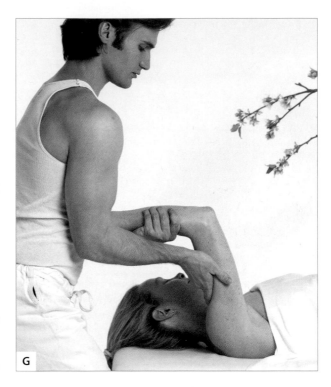

G

right hand. Put a gentle traction on her arm overhead before you walk it back around to her side and apply some more effleurage strokes from her hand to her shoulder and back to give her arm a feeling of connectedness. Those who engage in yoga or work out at a gym frequently have tight, sore triceps, and kneading them will feel really delicious.

4. OPEN THE CHEST WITH LONG AND SHORT STROKES

Placing your left hand on your partner's shoulder, apply effleurage across her upper chest and back for a few strokes. If her shoulders are lifted off the table because her pectoralis (upper chest) muscles are tight, spend extra time on that area with circular friction and lean into the effleurage strokes more to encourage length in the chest muscles.

5. REPEAT THE SEQUENCE ON THE RIGHT

Repeat the arm, shoulder, and chest massage on your partner's right side.

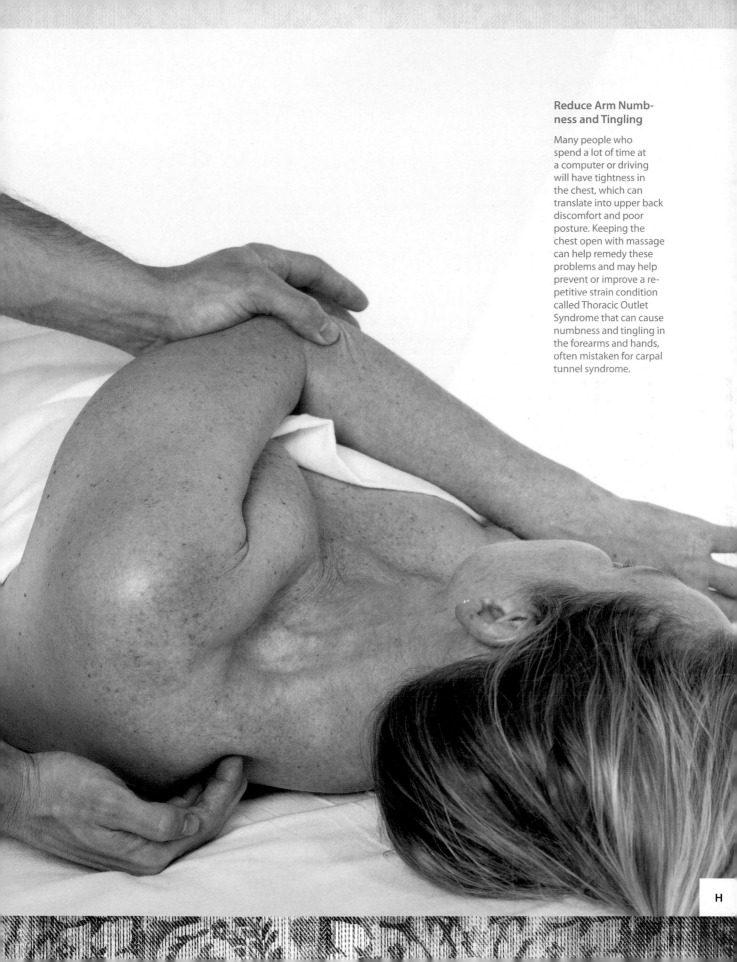

Reduce Arm Numbness and Tingling

Many people who spend a lot of time at a computer or driving will have tightness in the chest, which can translate into upper back discomfort and poor posture. Keeping the chest open with massage can help remedy these problems and may help prevent or improve a repetitive strain condition called Thoracic Outlet Syndrome that can cause numbness and tingling in the forearms and hands, often mistaken for carpal tunnel syndrome.

Supine Lower Body and Abdominal Sequence

When you massage your partner's feet, legs, thighs, and hips, you will find that she frequently is unaware of tightness and discomfort residing there from the demands of work or recreation. Increasing circulation to the lower extremities often reduces swelling and makes the limbs feel more awake and alive.

FREE THE HIPS

Use the leg as a lever to address the back of the pelvis and create a welcome feeling of freeing the hips.

Lift Legs to Roll Them Inward

Move to your partner's right leg and thigh. Notice whether her feet point roughly up at the ceiling or whether they are turned strongly out to the sides. If they turn significantly outward, reach under her waistline with your left hand, almost to the vertebral column, and under the broadest part of her hip with your right hand, palms up. Lift your fingers strongly upward and pull her pelvis toward you, which will roll her leg and thigh inward. Repeat at her hip and upper thigh, then at her thigh and leg, each time rotating her thigh and leg a little farther inward (photo A).

After you have completed these pulls, her foot should be less turned out and she will feel as though there is a pleasant openness in the posterior pelvis. Repeat the broadening action on her left side; then return to her right leg and thigh. This broadening helps to counteract the effects of sitting with legs crossed, which shortens the posterior hip muscles and can create tightness and discomfort in the hips and low back.

1. EFFLEURAGE AND PETRISSAGE FROM RIGHT TOES TO HIP

Perform several effleurage strokes with both hands from your partner's toes to her hip to spread lubricant and begin to palpate for tight areas. Stand at the side of the table with your hips facing the direction of your strokes and remember that your strokes toward her heart should be considerably firmer than those toward her feet. Stand at the side of the table near her thigh and knead her thigh muscles (quadriceps) with the full, firm palms of both hands, feeding the tissue back and forth from one hand to the other, lifting and squeezing rhythmically until you feel a softening of the quadriceps muscles.

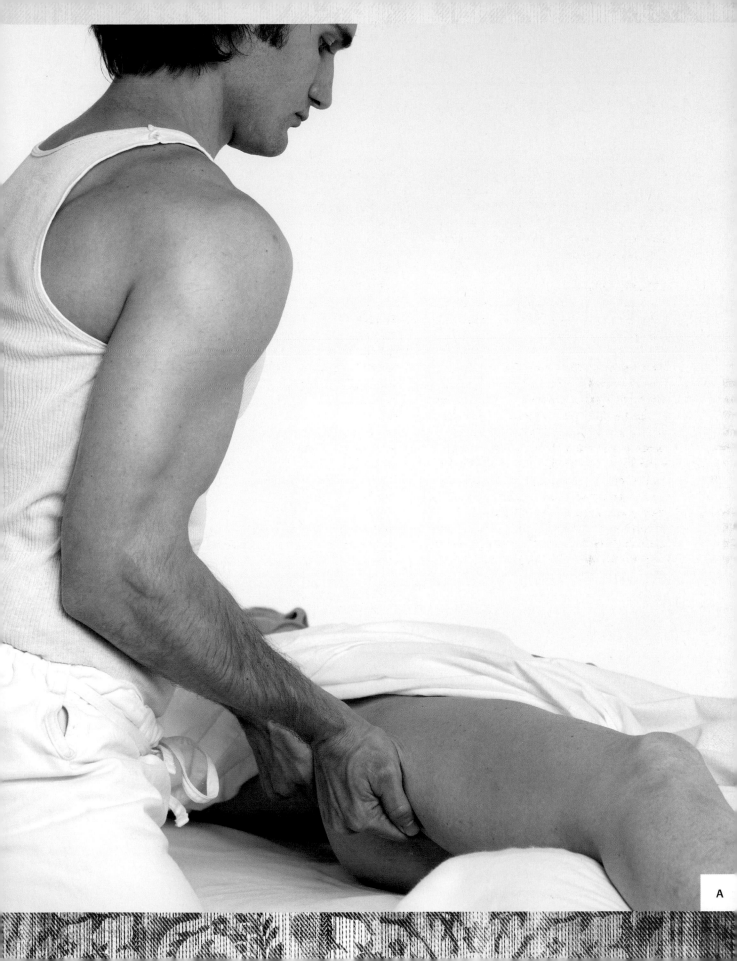

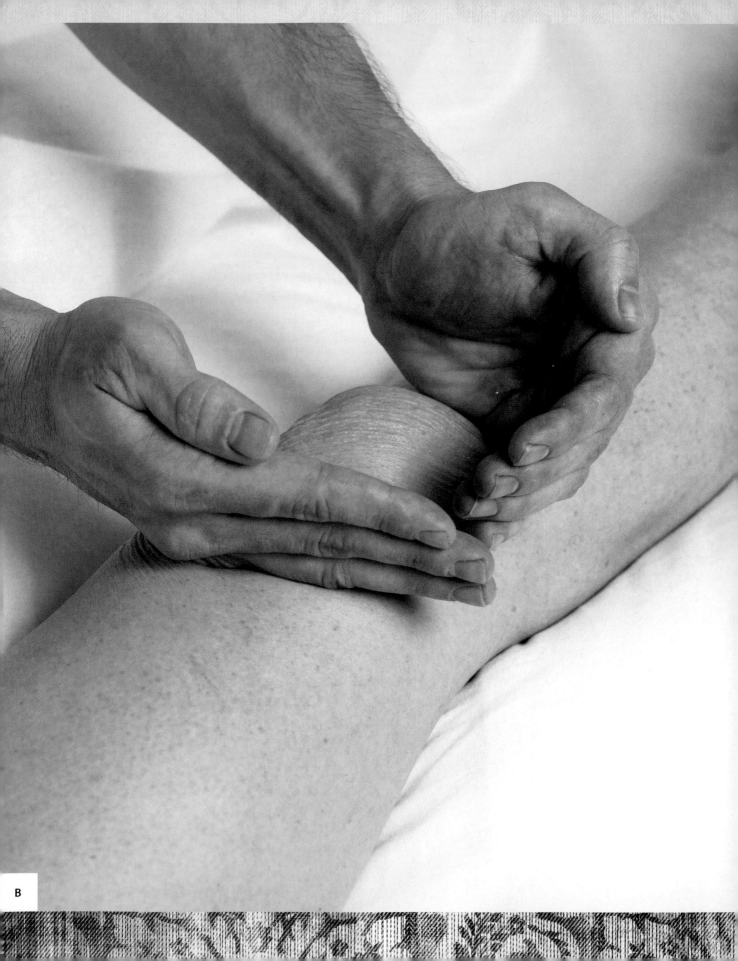

Lift, Shake, and Knead the Thigh

You may lift the muscles up and shake the tissue in place, which causes a vibration through the muscles. This is a movement the body can't "push back" against, so it relaxes muscles that may have difficulty letting go. Place your knee on the table next to your partner's lateral thigh to hold it in place as you apply pulling strokes on her medial thigh, up and down between her knee and groin. Remove your knee from the table and make vertical circles on her medial and lateral thigh, moving up and down between her knee and groin.

With each upward stroke that you use to lift the thigh muscles, you may pull your hands back toward you, making jostling motions with the thigh as you do so; like shaking the muscles, this movement relaxes muscles that may be holding tension from stair climbing or athletic activities.

Use Circular and Cross-Fiber Friction around the Knee

When you arrive at your partner's knee, use circular friction with your fingertips around her knee (**photo B**); then, facing the head of the table, perform cross-fiber friction with your thumbs just above her knee, with your thumbs crossing each other and forming circles just medial to her knee (**photo C**) using enough pressure to create some pinking of the skin around her knee. There are attachments of muscles at the medial knee that are often tight, and performing friction in the area can reduce knee discomfort.

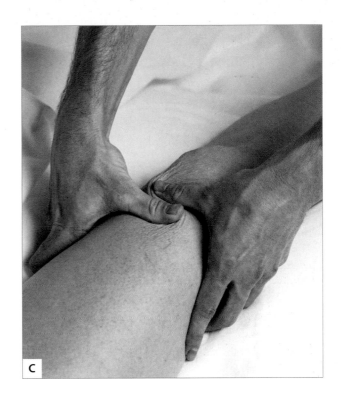

C

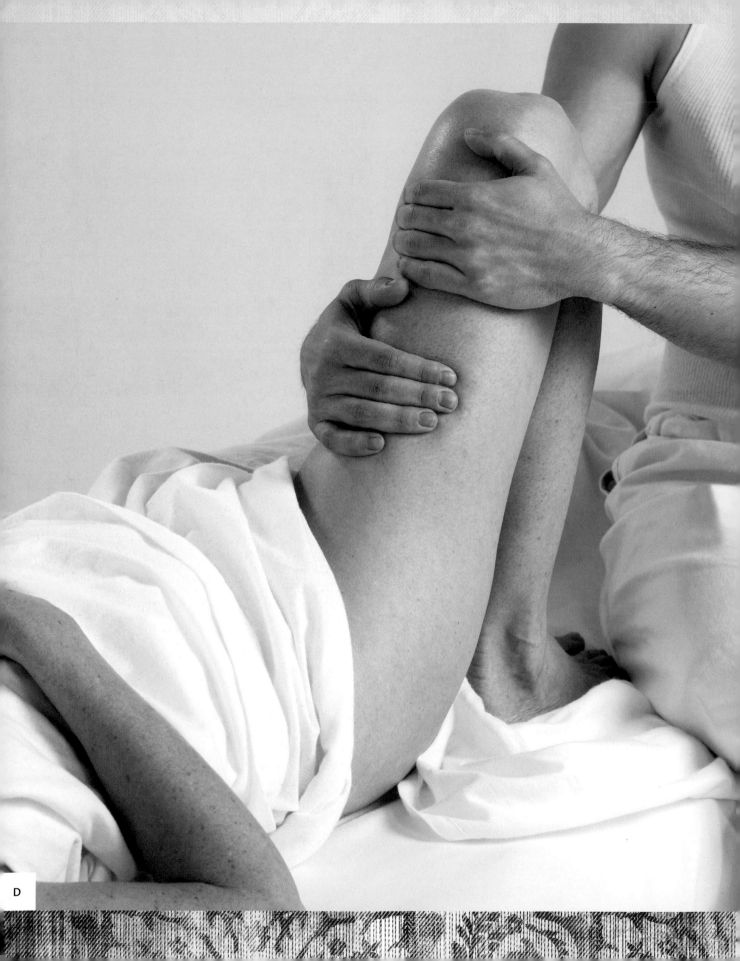

D

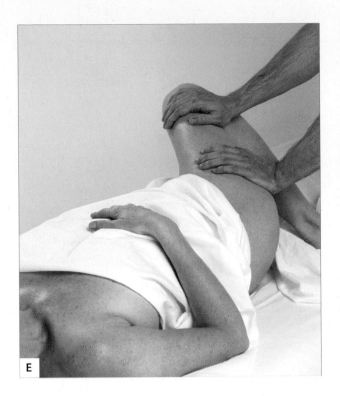

E

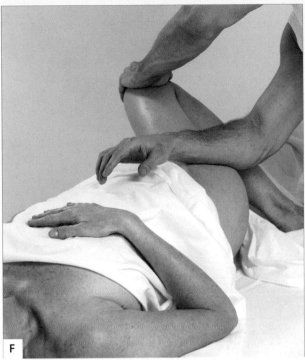

F

2. STRETCH THE BACK

With your partner's foot on the table, as close to her buttock as is comfortable for her, take a seat on the table just past her toes and wrap your arms around her thigh. Rock back with your whole torso, pulling her thigh toward you, to the natural stopping point of her stretch. Keep your hands in continuous contact with her thigh, allowing it to spring back torward her torso. Find her natural rhythm and flow with it, gradually gaining more movement, and allowing the knee to move medially and leterally with the pulls and rebounds **(photo D)**.

3. OPEN THE HIP BY ROCKING THE THIGH

Place your partner's foot on the table, with her heel as close to her buttocks as is comfortable, and rock her thigh gently and rhythmically away from you, with your knee on the table just past her toes to keep her foot from sliding down the table **(photo E)**. Just push her leg and thigh away; they will rebound back toward you at a rate that is her rhythmic pace. Try to keep the rocking fluid and don't allow her leg to rebound all the way back, but encourage more opening in the posterior hip. When you feel some loosening in the hip joint, use your right forearm to glide deeply from her lateral knee to her hip two or three times, leaning your body weight gently into the stroke **(photo F)**. Perform this broad stroke on the dense connective tissue on the lateral portion of the thigh to create a feeling of more space and length in the thigh.

Release Physical and Emotional Discomfort

Massaging around the hip joint will release hips that have become bound up from sitting too long, especially with the legs crossed, or from long commutes. Emotional discomfort can build up in the hips as well—note our language regarding situations that are "a pain in the butt."

Work Sensitively around the Hip

Still taking slack out of your partner's lateral thigh and hip by maintaining pressure with your left hand to hold the stretch over her left leg, use the fingers on your right hand to apply circular friction around the hip joint. Because many people are tender in the hips, you should work sensitively in the area, applying circular friction all the way around the lateral hip bone (the trochanter). The muscle attachments around the bone radiate out like spokes, and you may feel taut bands in the area, which will benefit greatly from additional circular and cross-fiber friction, as well as some compression.

4. PAY ATTENTION TO THE CALF, ANKLE, AND FOOT

Return your partner's leg and thigh to the table, performing a few superficial connecting effleurage (gliding) strokes on the entire length of her limb. Then with one hand on the medial side of her leg and the other on the lateral side, apply petrissage (lift, shake, and wring) strokes to the calf muscles followed by alternating hand-pushing strokes up her lower leg to her knee. Vigorously wring her ankle with both hands. From the end of the table, move into her foot with your thumbs on the medial arch. Milk her foot by squeezing one hand, then the other, on the medial and lateral sides, as you did with her hands. Then pull each toe with a little twist as you did with her fingers. All of these massage movements on the foot will help relieve foot pain from too much standing, fallen arches, or inadequate arch support in shoes.

5. REPEAT THE SEQUENCE ON THE LEFT LEG

Effleurage your partner's foot, leg, and thigh two or three times to give the entire limb a feeling of connectedness and repeat the lower extremity massage on the left side.

6. USE A LONGER CONTACT HOLD FOR THE ABDOMEN

Stand on the left side of the table and face your partner's abdomen. You may undrape her torso or give her a pillowcase to place over her breasts if she is either modest or chilly. Place your hands slowly and firmly, but without much weight, on her abdomen and offer a stationary contact hold.

Clockwise Circles and Pulls on the Abdomen

After you have held your hands immobile for two or three of your partner's breaths, begin a few clockwise circles around her abdomen with both hands (**photo G**). It is important to remember to always use a clockwise direction as it is the direction in which the contents of the intestines flow through the digestive tract. By following the natural direction, you may reduce symptoms of constipation. Petrissage the entire abdominal area, paying special attention to kneading slowly and calmly so as not to elicit ticklishness. Perform some strokes across your partner's belly, pushing toward the opposite side with one hand while the other hand pulls toward you, with your hands passing each other around the midline of her body. Be sure to start at the sides of her torso; you may use your forearms in addition to your hands for this stroke, and you may move up and down between your partner's pubic bone and her rib cage.

Warning! Ease into These Places

Although massage on every part of the body should begin with a brief contact hold to accustom the receiver to touch in the particular area, it is especially important in sensitive areas such as the abdomen, the side of the torso, the buttocks, and the feet. If you feel an abdominal pulse under your hands, move them from that area of the belly or lighten the pressure until you do not detect the pulse.

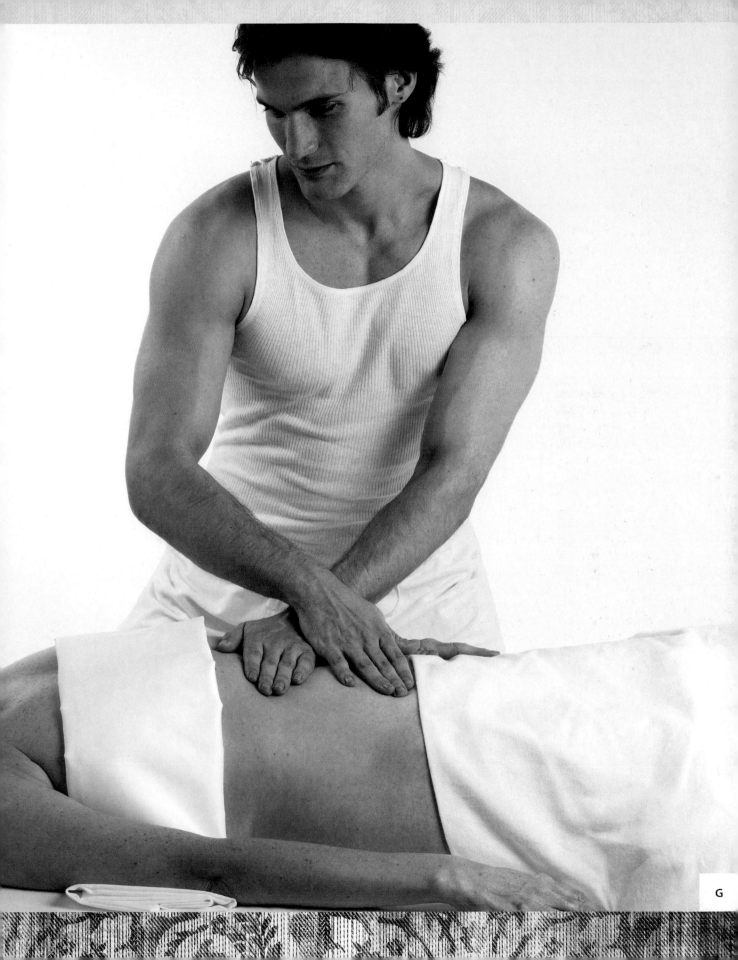

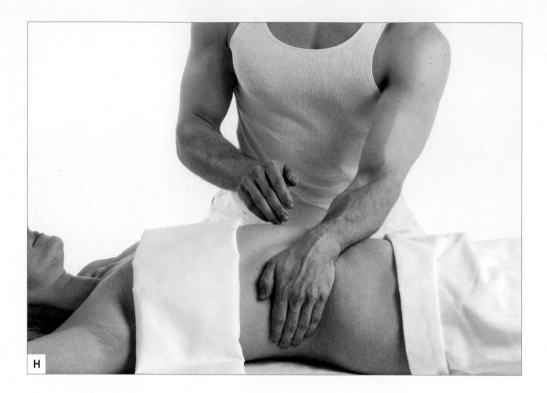

H

Alternate Hand-Pulling Strokes along the Torso

Reach across your partner's torso and using both hands apply alternating hand-pulling strokes from her hip to her armpit; brace your thighs against the side of the table for stability, exerting firm pressure as you bring your hands toward you **(photos H and I)**. This pulling stroke twists the torso and stretches a number of the back muscles in a way that can help relieve some low back pain. If she especially likes the twisting motion of the pulling stroke, place her arm across her chest and begin again to alternate pulling strokes from her hip, moving up her torso and continuing all the way up the back of her shoul-

der. Respect the amount of stretch in her back, recognizing where you meet any resistance to the stretch and make sure the stretch continues to be comfortable. When you have your left arm and hand behind her shoulder and your right arm and hand at her middle back, simply hold the stretch for a few breaths and release slowly as you reverse the twist and return her back to the table.

A Contact Hold before Transitioning to Prone (Face Down)

Place one hand on your partner's upper chest and the other on her abdomen, over her navel. Hold for three or four of her breaths and then have her turn to a prone (face-down) position.

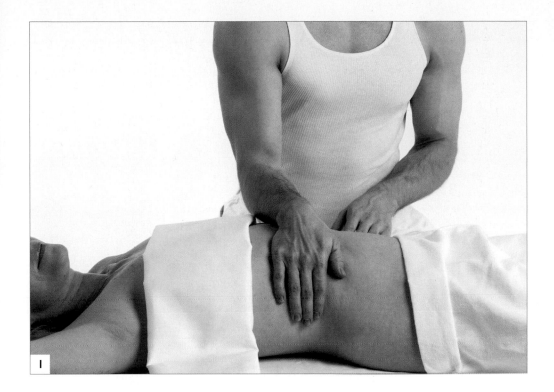

I

The Benefits of Swedish Massage

- Relieves muscular soreness, fatigue, discomfort, and tension
- Tones weak muscles; increases muscle length and flexibility
- Reduces excessive scar formation and adhesions
- Promotes healing of fractures
- Reduces the surface dimpling of cellulite
- Promotes relaxation and reduces anxiety, depression, discomfort, and stress
- Improves the balance of hormones and neurotransmitters in the body
- Improves circulation, nourishing and oxygenating the cells and removing waste
- Increases platelets as well as red and white blood cells
- Decreases blood pressure and reduces edema (swelling)
- Improves lung function and decreases asthma attacks
- Stimulates digestion and relieves constipation
- Enhances fertility, decreases menopausal and PMS symptoms, and assists in labor, delivery, and lactation
- Enhances intimacy and connection

Prone Sequence:
Loosen and Lengthen the Back, Legs, and Hips

The hamstrings and calf muscles—chronically tight in many people, especially if they are athletic—are more accessible in the prone position. In addition, it is possible to reduce the appearance of cellulite on the hips and posterior thighs by massaging them.

FACE DOWN COMFORT MEASURES PAY ATTENTION TO COMFORT

The recipient will be more comfortable in the prone position if you set up the table carefully.

Position a Pillow beneath the Ankles

Place a pillow under your partner's ankles as she lies face down on the table. This allows her feet to hang over the edge of the pillow rather than being strongly plantar-flexed on the surface of the table.

1. LENGTHEN AND KNEAD THE LEG

Undrape your partner's left leg and thigh and effleurage the length of her leg from the sole of her foot to her buttock, spreading lubricant. As with all lubricant-spreading strokes, start with light pressure and gradually increase the pressure with repetitions of strokes. After a few full effleurage strokes, move to your partner's thigh and begin petrissage strokes there, lifting and squeezing the tissue and feeding it back and forth from one hand to the other hand. As you feel her muscles begin to soften, you may use the backs of your fingers or all of your fingers together to perform deeper effleurage strokes from just above her knee to her sit bones; these strokes will follow the hamstrings, a group of muscles which tend to be tight and frequently contribute to low back pain by pulling the pelvis down. See if you can feel the fibers as they run from medial and lateral to her knee all the way up to her lower buttock crease. Applying deep effleurage slowly and leaning in will gradually encourage length in the hamstring muscles.

2. IRON THE HAMSTRINGS

You may also use your right forearm with your palm facing down and your elbow pointing toward your partner's right leg to slowly iron out the hamstring muscles, moving slowly (photo A). If you want to reduce some of the tension in the hamstrings while you massage them, lift your partner's foot at the ankle with your right hand so that it is above her knee and make several long strokes on her thigh with your left hand. Exercise caution with your pressure. Tight hamstrings are tender hamstrings. Be sure to ease into pressure very gradually.

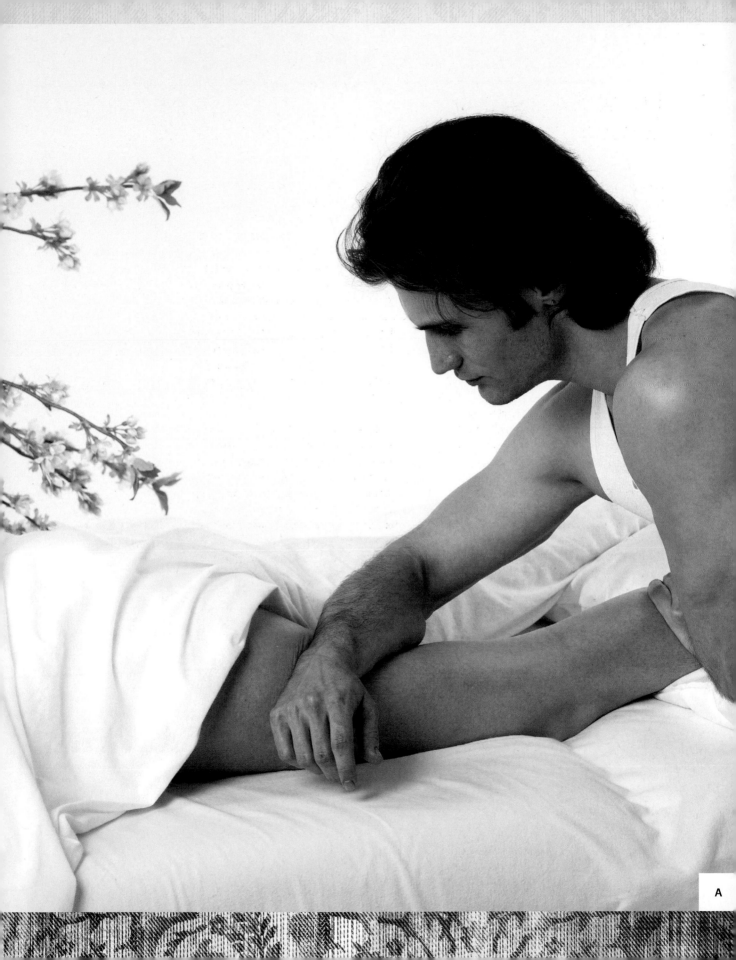

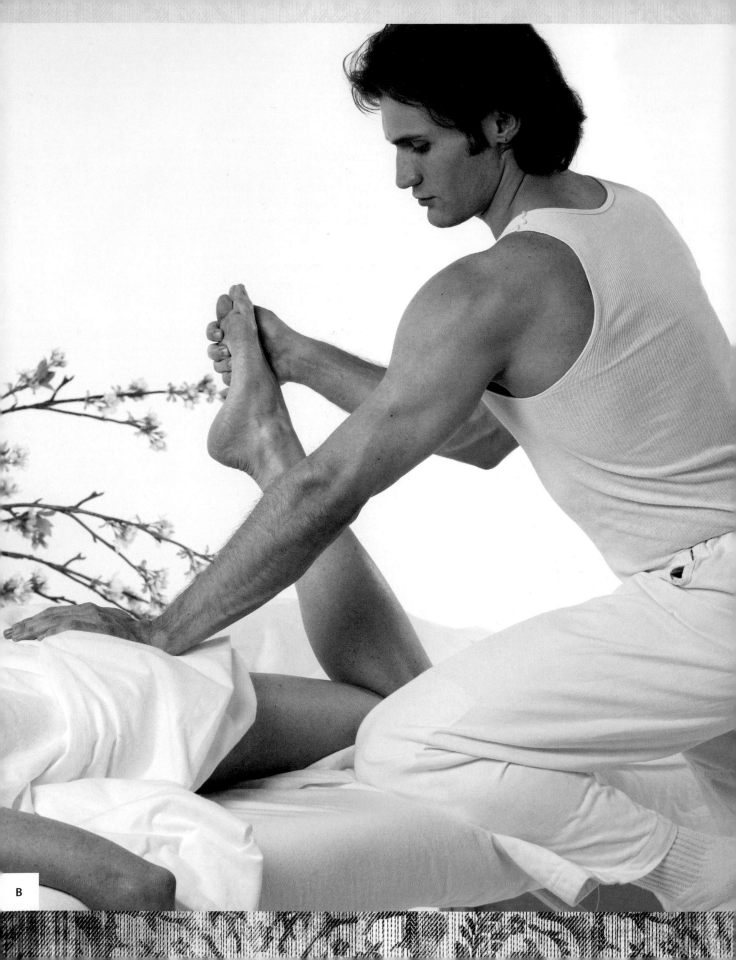

3. FIND THE RANGE OF MOTION FOR THE LOWER LEG AND FOOT

Hold your partner's left foot with your palm facing up under the top of her foot and your fingers curved around the ball of her foot. Place your left hand on her sacrum and press down firmly; this will reduce the likelihood of her hip lifting as you perform the stretch. With a quick rotation of your wrist away from yourself, flick your partner's heel away **(photo B)**. It will return to a neutral position at its own rate, establishing the rhythm for repeated heel flicks, during which you may rotate her foot and leg closer to and farther away from her buttocks, as well as closer to and farther away from yourself. These range-of-motion circles for the lower leg help create a lot of movement in the calf muscle. Because these muscles are often tight and tender, this indirect method of loosening them may be more comfortable for your partner than more direct pressure.

4. STIMULATE CIRCULATION IN THE CALF

Standing at the left side of the table near the lower leg, place your partner's leg back onto the table and pillow and petrissage her calf muscles just as you did her thigh. You may also lift the tissue and shake it as you did with her hamstrings. Move closer to her foot and apply alternating hand-pushing strokes from above her ankle almost to her knee. This stimulates circulation in the lower leg. Then clasp your fingers together, as if in prayer, and squeeze the side of her calves with the heels of your hands, bringing your hands together off the back of her leg as you gradually move toward her knee with the strokes. Apply some light effleurage strokes to her entire leg and thigh, making figure eights, with half of the figure eight on her lower leg and half on her thigh, fluidly connecting the limb. Remember to concentrate the strokes so that circulation flows toward the heart!

5. CIRCLE THE HEELS, STROKE THE ARCH

When you return to your partner's ankle after a few repetitions, circle the heels of your thumbs on the sides of her heels, from the ankle bones to the sole at the heel. Not only will this feel great on her heels, but it will also reinvigorate your hands. Hold the dorsal surface of her foot in your right hand, which can be resting on the pillow, and use the backs of your fingers (left hand) to make an arching stroke along the medial arch of her foot. With your thumbs side by side, apply some deep strokes from the ball of her foot to the front of her heel.

6. REPEAT THE SEQUENCE ON THE RIGHT

Hold your partner's foot between your hands for a couple of breaths before repeating the foot, leg, and thigh massage on her right limb.

Prone Upper Body Sequence:
Smoothing out the Back, Hip, and Legs

This sequence creates length in the postural muscles of the back, which continuously hold us upright, and increases flexibility in the back, shoulders, and hips. This is an area most of us cannot reach to rub for ourselves, so the back is especially appreciative of targeted attention. Almost everyone has areas of tension and discomfort in some region of the back.

1. GLIDE OVER THE BACK, HIPS, AND SHOULDERS

Stand at the head of the table with your partner's back undraped. Spread lubricant on her back with several effleurage strokes. Keep your weight evenly on your hands, from your fingertips to the heels of your hands, and lean in to glide to each side of the vertebral column from her shoulders to her hips, gradually increasing from light to moderate pressure as you repeat strokes. When you arrive at her hips, spread your hands apart and make a spreading stroke across her upper hips; then bring your hands in toward the center of her back before pulling them back toward you, broadening at her upper back and making a spreading stroke all the way around her shoulder joint before returning to her upper mid-back. Apply several of these long hourglass-shaped, integrated strokes, which will give your partner a sense of length through her entire back and shoulders.

2. ALTERNATE HAND-PUSHING STROKES ALONG ONE SIDE OF THE SPINE

Scoop your partner's upper trapezius muscle toward the ceiling with your right hand as you begin alternating hand-pushing strokes down the right side of her back (**photo A**), moving down along the side of the table as you apply the strokes. When both of your hands have arrived at her waist, turn and face her head and repeat the pushing strokes back up toward her shoulders (**photo B**).

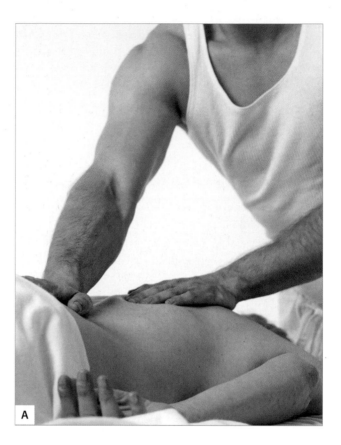

A

Knead the Opposite Side of the Back

Reach across to the left side of your partner's back and petrissage the muscles between her spine and her left side, lifting and squeezing the tissue and feeding it back and forth between your hands. The reason to petrissage on the opposite side of the back is to keep your wrists in a neutral position; it can be very hard on your hands to hyperextend your wrists to knead the side of the back closest to you. Keep your thumbs and forefingers of both hands spread wide apart and "aim" the tissue toward the C shape of your opposite hand, moving side to side as you petrissage.

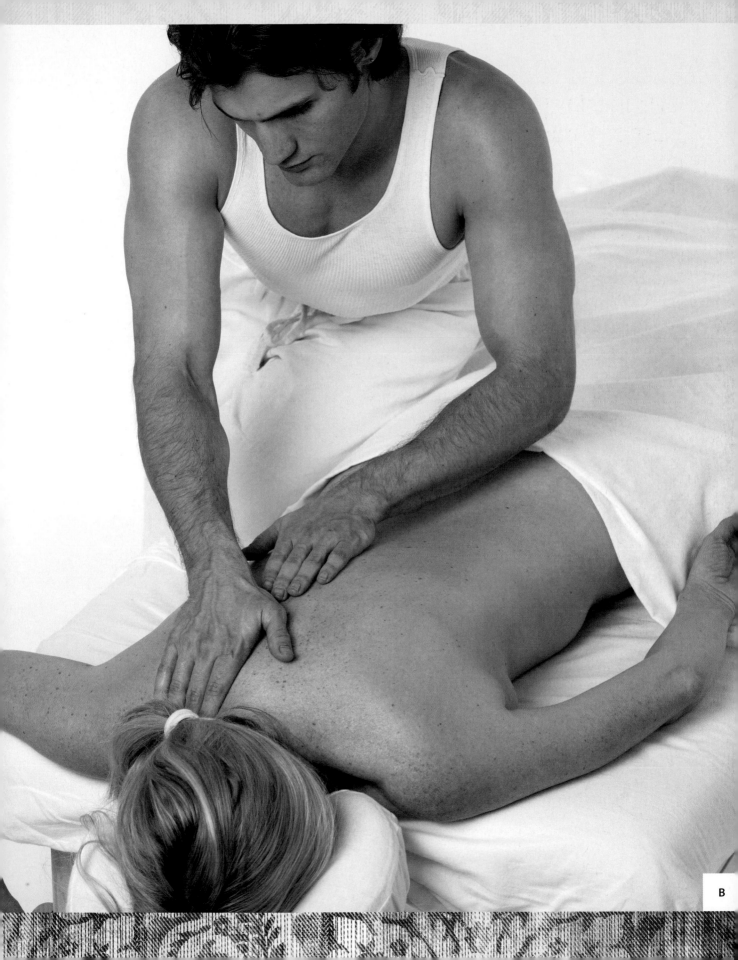

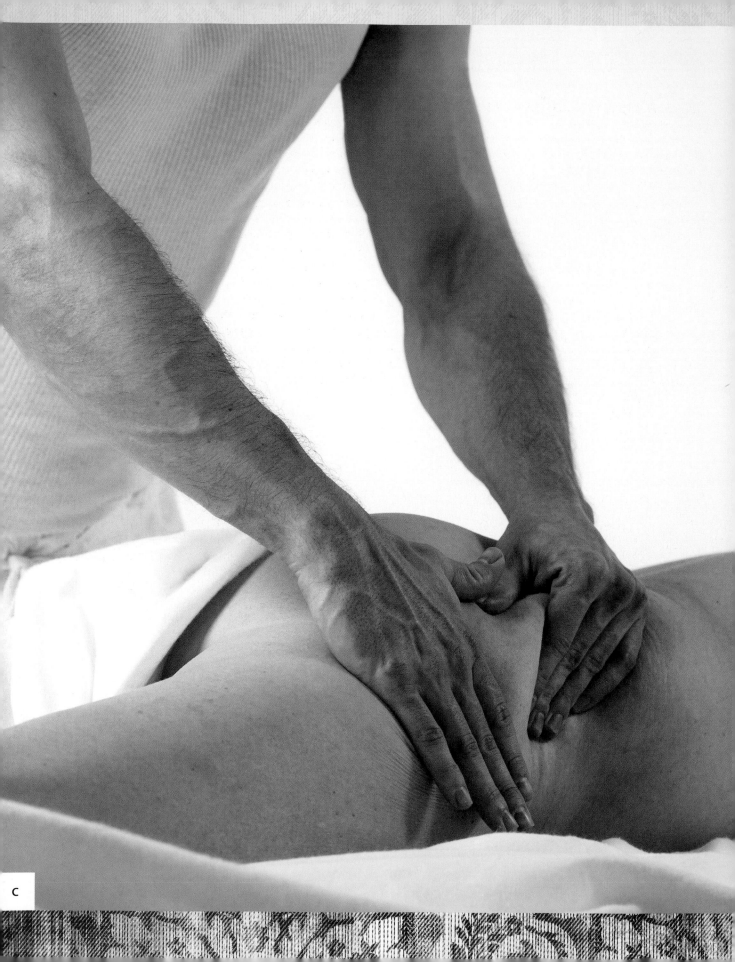

C

3. ADD FRICTION AND VIBRATION FOR THE GLUTES AND SACRUM

You may also undrape your partner's buttock on the side of her back you are petrissaging and continue kneading into the gluteal muscles sensitively **(photo C)**; frequently, there are tight areas in the gluteal area, and kneading this area can help reduce discomfort and tightness in the hip and low back. (Everything is, after all, connected.) Place your fingertips on her sacrum, the bony area about the size of your hand just below the middle waistline, and apply circular friction on the bone, feeling for the bone's indentations. Then, extending your arm at the shoulder, elbow, and wrist, create vibration that starts at your shoulder, moves down through your arm and hand, and vibrates deeply into her sacrum and the muscles that lie beneath it. Often, applying vibration on the sacrum will feel to the receiver like having a deep itch scratched.

4. PETRISSAGE THE UPPER SHOULDERS

Move toward your partner's head and petrissage the upper trapezius muscles of both shoulders again, drawing your flattened fingers toward the heels of your hand, stabilized against the uppermost part of her back, or stabilizing your fingers in front and pushing the heels of your hands toward your fingers. Find out which movement your partner prefers or throw in a few repetitions of each. You may also perform both actions at once, squeezing with your fingers and the heels of your hands. Again, keep your entire palm on the tissue so that it doesn't pinch. You may also apply the same kind of back-and-forth petrissage you performed on the left side of her back on her upper-right shoulder before you move to the left side of her head to repeat the back massage.

Knead Like a Baker

The back can be a challenging place to petrissage, as it is a relatively broad and flat expanse, and you must keep your palms fairly flat on the muscles, lifting with your palms as well as your extended fingers so that this move does not feel pinchy. By doing this correctly, you will develop hand muscles that bakers tend to develop.

Swedish Massage Has Roots in Rome

In the Western world, massage dates back as far as the ancient Greeks and Romans. The widely acknowledged father of modern medicine, Hippocrates, and his own teacher, Herodicus, wrote on the value of physical manipulation of the body's joints and muscles and the therapeutic value of exercise. These texts were studied during the Middle Ages and the Renaissance in Europe.

Pehr Henrik Ling, a Swedish physiologist and gymnastics instructor, was acquainted with these ancient works. He developed a system he called Swedish gymnastics, by which passive and active movements and specific massage strokes were used to reduce discomforts and abnormalities. Between 1813 and 1839, he taught his Swedish Movement System, later to be called Swedish massage, to a large number of physicians and nonmedical students who spread his ideas widely through Europe and elsewhere. In 1856, Drs. George and Charles Taylor, brothers who had studied the Swedish Movement System in Europe, imported it to the United States.

Create Space between the Shoulder Blades

Returning to the head of the table, place your left hand over your right hand and apply a few slow effleurage strokes on the left side of your partner's upper back from the base of her neck to the medial border of her scapula (photo D). You are pushing the muscle fibers away from you and lengthening them from the spine. The direction of this short stroke is about forty-five degrees downward to follow the fiber direction of the rhomboid muscles, which are often sore. Repeat the stroke slowly a few times, moving a little downward at each stroke so that the last one ends at the lowest point of the scapula. Repeat on the right side.

Find the Range of Motion in the Shoulder

Standing on your partner's left side, hold her left upper arm in your left palm loosely just above the elbow, with her forearm and hand hanging down toward the floor. Lean back and rock from foot to foot, swinging her arm from side to side and putting some traction on her upper arm and upper back muscles. Moving the limb as you stretch the muscles tends to confuse them into lengthening more than they would otherwise. Take your partner's right wrist in your right hand, still holding above her elbow with your left hand, and lift her entire forearm up slightly; then rotate it medially and laterally. Perform this range of motion for her shoulder slowly so that you can feel when you are approaching the end point of the stretch in each direction and don't exceed those natural limitations; just work the edge, which will gradually increase as you make several rotations. Check in with your partner about whether you are remaining within her comfortable range of motion.

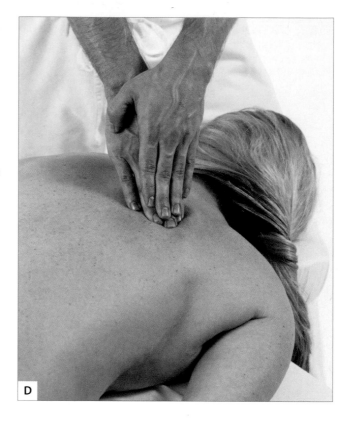

D

Jostle the "Chicken Wings"

Place your partner's arm on the table, with her elbow flexed and her hand near her waistline. Put your knee on the table just past her hand so that her arm will remain in place. Reach under her shoulder with your left hand and hold her upper arm in your right palm. With loose and floppy hands, lift her shoulder and arm alternately (photo E); this move is affectionately termed chicken wings to give you an idea of the action you are aiming for.

Try to keep the movement fluid rather than jerky and honor the natural limits in range of motion; you will feel a change when your partner allows full freedom of movement in her shoulder, elbow, and wrist. This movement actually helps free up the upper chest muscles as well.

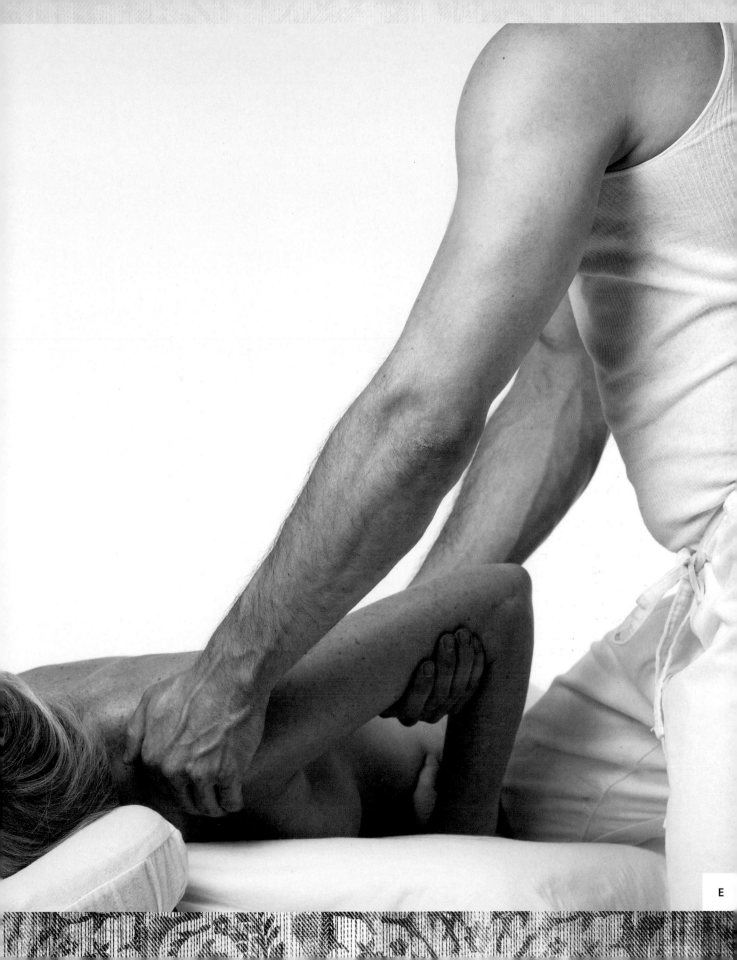

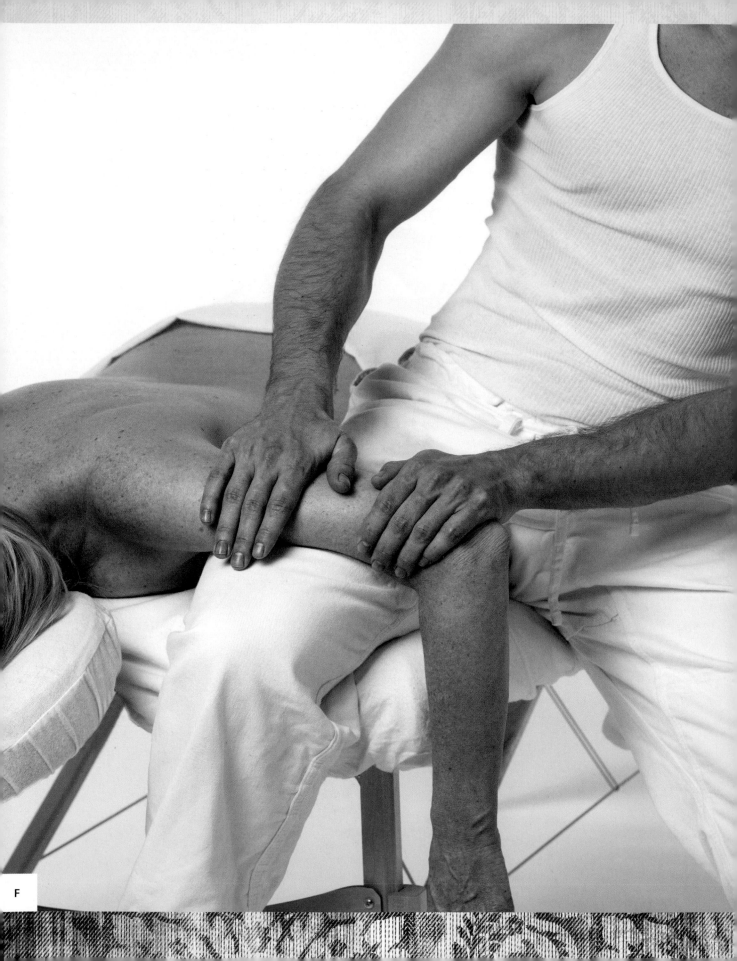

5. ROLL THE UPPER ARM

Remove your knee from the table and lifting your partner's upper arm with your left hand, sit on the front-left corner of the table with her upper arm over your thigh. Roll the muscles with both of your palms back and forth and as you press down on her upper arm, lean out to your left (**photo F**). This will stretch the "root" of the arm within the shoulder and will noticeably broaden the shoulder, releasing the muscles that become tight in the upper back, chest, and shoulder. When you feel you have loosened her shoulder as much as it seems inclined to let go, hold her left arm in your palm and return to a standing position, placing her arm on the table by her side.

6. BEAT, SLAP, AND TAP THE BACK

Effleurage your partner's entire back, using long, hourglass-shaped strokes again to integrate the entire back, after working specific parts of her back, hips, and shoulders. With one hand on each side of her spine and avoiding areas where bones such as the scapulas are close to the surface, begin to apply tapotement, or tapping to her back, with alternating hands. Using the sides of your fists beat up and down her back. Follow with hacking strokes, the kind you always saw trainers in old movies performing on athletes, using the ulnar sides of your hands with your fingers extended. Next, apply tapotement with your cupped palms; this makes a very satisfying sound, similar to the clopping of horses' hooves. Slapping tapotement is next, followed by tapping with your fingertips all over the back. Tapotement increases circulation and stimulates the nervous system. It confuses the muscles into releasing further, and if your partner has fallen asleep during the massage, tapotement is likely to wake her up.

7. SLOW TO A COMFORTABLE HALT WITH ROCKING

Always follow tapotement with effleurage to "make nice." Gradually slow your strokes up and down your partner's back and very lightly bring your alternating hand's fingertips up her back, neck, and the back of her head to end the back massage. Come to her side and place one hand on her upper back and the other at the hip nearest to you. Gently ease into rocking her back and hips away from you and find her rhythm as her body comes back from the rocking, keeping the movement fluid and nurturing, like rocking a baby. Gradually rock more slowly and with smaller motions until your hands are resting on her still back. Maintain this contact hold for at least three of her breaths before removing your hands and thanking her for honoring you by trusting her body to your hands.

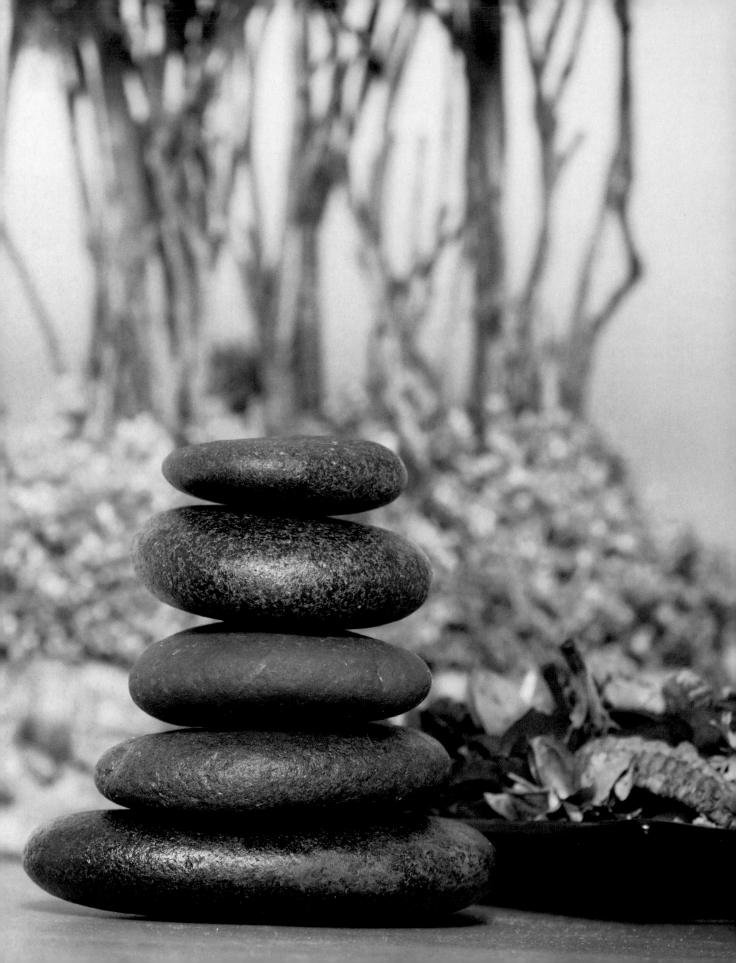

CHAPTER 2

Hot Stone Massage Melts Muscle Tension

With hot stone massage, basalt stones are heated in water and placed at specific locations on the body or moved on the skin. Marble stones cooled in ice water are frequently used in hot stone sessions both for contrast and for the therapeutic value of cooling tissues.

Hot stones may be integrated into Asian massage forms such as Thai and shiatsu by moving them along the meridian or sen lines. They can be used with reflexology by stimulating the points on the feet or hands; with lomi lomi to create heated flowing strokes; and most commonly, with Swedish massage as a tool. Ideally, hot stones are used in such a seamless way that they blend into whatever form is being used, adding the comforting, grounding, therapeutic, and penetrating qualities of heat.

The Pressure and Strokes of Hot Stone Massage

The heat of the stones helps to melt muscle tension, so you may want to use less pressure than you would use with your hands. Also, you do not have the sensitivity of your hands when you are performing strokes with stones, so it is best to massage with them more superficially. In general, most of the strokes and sequences used in Swedish massage (see chapter 1) work with hot stones. Become comfortable and practiced with the Swedish sequence before adding hot stones to it.

You may lean in with the stones and feel as though you are ironing out the knots and tight areas. At any time, you may put down one or both stones and continue with the basic Swedish strokes with your warmed hands. For instance, you may hold your partner's hand in one of your hands and use a stone in your other hand to effleurage down his arm toward his elbow, or you may spread the palm of your partner's hand with one hand and use a small working stone to apply friction to his palm with the other hand. Remember that heavy people require no more pressure than thin people; in fact, they may be more sensitive to pressure.

KNOW YOUR STROKES

Use enough strokes in each area for your partner to relax into the stroke without becoming annoyed by it. Generally speaking, three to five strokes tend to feel good, but a dozen would probably irritate.

Effleurage—Using the flat palm with fingers together, you glide away from your torso with neutral (not flexed or hyperextended) wrists. Effleurage strokes may be performed by one or both hands or with forearms in some areas of the body.

Petrissage— With the palm in full contact with the skin, you knead, lift, and squeeze the muscle tissue. This is a difficult stroke to perform with stones in your palms; you may want to put the stone down and use your hands.

For more on strokes, see chapter 9.

Warning!
Hot Stone Massage Is Dangerous for Some

Anyone who has impaired sensitivity to heat and cold, such as a person with diabetic neuropathy, is not a good candidate to receive hot stone massage; it is of critical importance that your partner be able to accurately assess if a stone is too hot.

Any inflammation, such as bursitis, rheumatoid arthritis, lupus, or autoimmune disorders that produce symptoms of redness, heat, and swelling, contraindicate the use of hot stones, but using cold stones may feel refreshing and may help reduce inflammation.

Use of hot stones should be avoided for those with significant cardiovascular disease such as arteriosclerosis, uncontrolled high blood pressure, a recent heart attack, blood clots (thrombosis), or multiple strokes, since heat increases circulation and might overtax the circulatory system or cause a clot to move through the system, which can be very dangerous.

Multiple sclerosis, Parkinson's disease, and skin irritation symptoms may be intensified by application of hot stones. It is inadvisable to bring a pregnant woman's core temperature above its normal level, as damage to the fetus may occur, so the use of many or large placement stones is contraindicated during pregnancy, although limited use of hot stones as tools is acceptable.

When in doubt about whether the use of hot stones is appropriate for your partner, it may be wise to obtain the approval of your partner's physician.

Young children are often so sensitive to heat that a warm stone session would be more appropriate for them than a hot stone massage. Some elderly people may lack the sensitivity to feel when a stone might be burning them, and their skin can be fragile, so warm stones would be a better choice for them as well.

An Affinity for Stones

As you prepare your stones, you are taking the first step in developing a relationship with them. Some people sense differences in the energy of different stones, but even if you don't, you will learn which stones fit your hands well and begin to develop an affinity for particular stones.

Purchase the Materials

Hot stone massage involves the expense of purchasing stones, a heating unit, and other implements and requires more maintenance and cleanup than most other forms of massage, but its benefits outweigh the cost and inconvenience.

The stones most commonly used for hot stone massage are unpolished natural basalt stones available from many suppliers. It is a good idea to purchase stones from a reputable provider rather than finding river rocks yourself, as the suppliers make sure the stones they sell are basalt and therefore are unlikely to crack or break when

they are heated. For hot stone massage, you will require the following, at a minimum:

• Ten to twelve small, flat placement "toe stones"

• Eight to twelve small palm-working stones (about 1.5–2" x 3–3.5" [3.8–5.1 x 7.6–8.9 cm])

• Eight to twelve mid-size palm-working stones (about 2.5–3" x 4" [6.4–7.6 x 10.2 cm])

• Four to eight large placement stones (about 3.5" x 5" [8.9 x 12.7 cm])

You will find contact information for suppliers of stones in the Resources section of this book. Some forms of hot stone massage use polished gemstones in the colors of the chakras to place on those positions (see the "Chakra Sequence" section in chapter 4), and if you enjoy working with stones energetically, you may want to add some of these stones to your collection. Suppliers also have stone tools, such as pointed stones and polished marble stones for cold use, and over time you may want to collect some of these to vary your hot stone massage abilities.

WASH, DRY, OIL, AND BAKE THE STONES

When you receive your stones, wash them in warm water with dishwashing liquid, rinse them, and allow them to dry. Then lightly oil them with a non-nut-based oil, such as safflower, canola, or olive oil; this is because some people are allergic to nut oil. After you have oiled the stones, place them in a 180°F (82°C) oven for two or three hours or bake them on top of a woodstove. This process is like seasoning a cast-iron pan, filling in and smoothing out the pores in the stones. Your stones are now ready to be placed in an electric skillet (see "Setting Up the Session") with water and used for massage.

Many companies that sell stones also sell hot-stone heating units, which are essentially electric roasters. An electric skillet is less expensive than a roaster, heats the stones more quickly, and because it is shallower, reduces the likelihood you will burn yourself on the edge as you remove stones from the unit. Hot stones are never heated in a microwave but are always heated in water, which conducts a set amount of heat quickly and evenly.

Setting Up the Session

You may already have the other accessories you'll need, such as several hand towels, ideally in light colors or white, a handkerchief, a meat thermometer, an optional eye pillow, and a pitcher. You will need a table on which to place your skillet, towels, pitcher, and lubricant.

LUBRICATE STONES

Many people feel that oil is the best lubricant to use with stones, but any relatively slick massage lotion will work as well. Lotion will not build up on your stones if you wash them after each use, so the type of lubricant is really a personal preference. You may want to include some essential oils with the oil or massage lubricant you are using, such as lavender for relaxation. Orange or sandalwood may be used as a muscle relaxant or soothing agent. Use essential oil in your lubricants sparingly; the heat of the stones delivers the properties of the oils more strongly, so a drop or two in your oil should be plenty. You may place oil or lubricant in one or two conveniently placed bowls, or you may want to get a lotion dispenser that you can wear in a holster for dispensing lubricant; you'll have your hands full with the stones.

BE SAFE AND SECURE

The space where you set up to do hot stone massage can have any kind of flooring, but if the floor is tile, hardwood, or vinyl, you will need to place a rug that is a couple of feet (about 60–90 cm) wider than the massage table in each dimension in the space. This will muffle the sound of any stones you drop or that your partner knocks off the table during a session. There is nothing quite like the loud crack of a stone hitting a hard floor to disrupt relaxation!

Try Powder If Your Partner Is Sensitive to Oil

In Japanese hot stone massage, polished stones that are very smooth and slick are used without any lubrication or with a fine powder such as corn starch. If your partner is sensitive to oils or finds that oils promote acne, you can try powder as a lubricant.

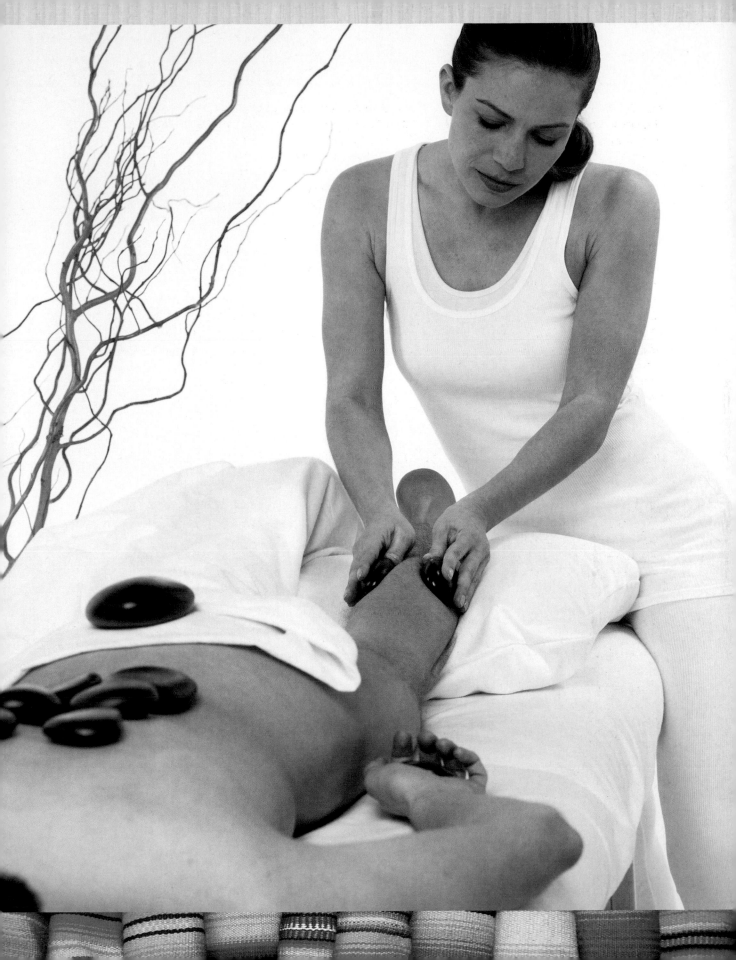

Place your stone table close to an electrical outlet; you do not want to risk tripping over an extension cord while giving a hot stone massage. The stone table should be at the side of the massage table, about three feet (91 cm) away, so that you can avoid moving a stone over your partner's face or head when you are placing it or removing it from his body. Stones and your hands may be wet or slick with oil and dropping one on your partner's head or face certainly will not contribute to his relaxation!

HEAT THE STONES

Place the electric skillet on the table, with a light-colored hand towel or thick dish towel in the skillet, covering the entire bottom and partway up the sides of the pan. Using a light-colored towel will make it easier to see and select the particular stone you want to use as you are massaging. Place your stones on their edges, lining them up in whatever order is logical to you. Place the little toe stones in the handkerchief and leave the ends of the handkerchief out of the water.

About fifteen minutes before you plan to use your stones, fill the skillet with about 2 inches (5.1 cm) of water and turn the skillet to a warm setting; then place the meat thermometer in the water so that you can read the temperature without moving it. Have the skillet lid on the pan while you are heating the stones, but once they reach their target temperature of 115°F–120°F (46°C–49°C), remove the cover for the duration of the hot stone session. Refill the pitcher with cold water and have it close at hand; it will serve to cool down your stones if they become too hot during a session. Place at least four hand towels close by, with one spread on the table to receive the stones you may not want to return to the skillet. Having a towel in the skillet and on the table will muffle the sounds the stones would make when placed on metal or wood. Some people like to have a slotted spoon to remove stones from the water.

Your best thermometers are your hands, at least at the beginning of a session. When you remove a stone from the water, it should be almost too hot to hold. However, a good guideline is that you should be able to comfortably hold a stone in your hand for more than five seconds. As you handle the hot stones during the massage, your hands will become desensitized to the heat to some degree.

The temperature of the stones in the skillet may change during the time you are massaging, so be sure to have towels ready in case you pick up a stone that's too hot to handle. It's best to have the stones a little too hot to place on your partner's body; you will gradually learn to manage your stones by removing ones from the pan you will be using in a few minutes to reach a comfortable temperature by the time you need them. Stones that you will be using in your hands may be hotter than those which will be stationary on your partner's body. Learning your individual stones' heat-holding qualities and your heating element's characteristics comes with practice and will help you maintain a graceful flow in a hot stone session.

COOL STONES FOR USE WITH ICE WATER

If you want to use some cool marble stones, you may place them in a shallow dish with ice water or water with ice cubes on the stone table. Alternatively, you may place them on the windowsill of the room where you are working in the winter and they will usually feel cool enough. To avoid dripping cold water if you use a bowl of ice water, place the cold stones on a hand towel before transferring them to your partner's body. Have your oil or lubricant conveniently placed to dip your hands into it or dispense it one-handed from a lotion dispenser.

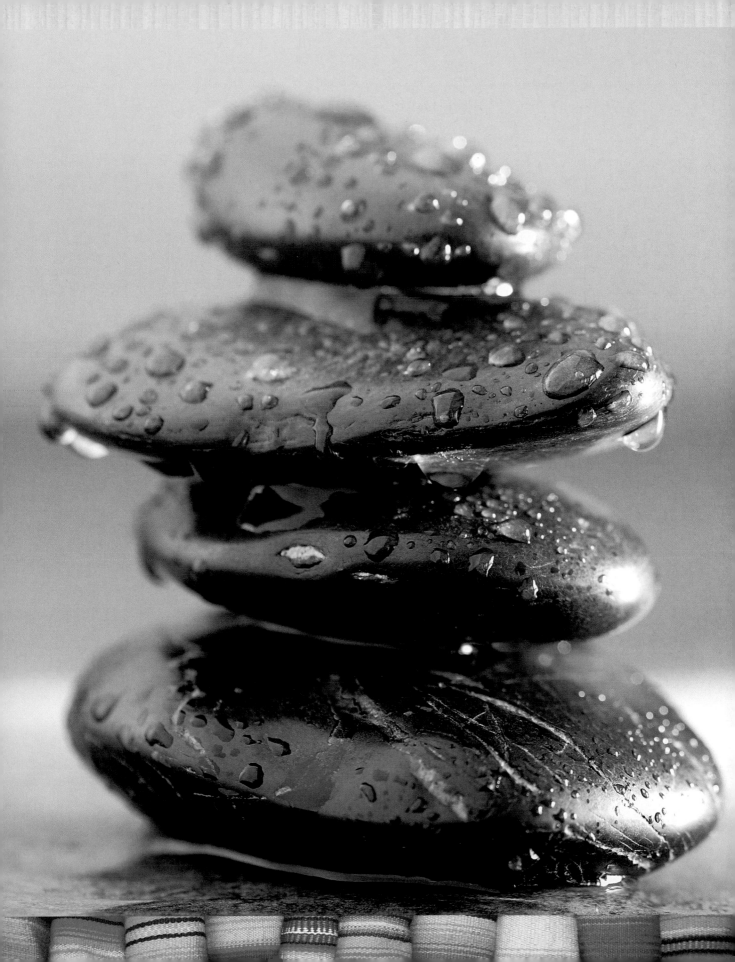

Placing Stones (Supine Sequence):
Anchoring the Body

A spa-type hot stone massage consists primarily of placing the stones on energy centers of the body. The weight and heat of the stones can have a profound effect even without the additional use of stones as tools in your hands. Rub all stones between your palms before you place them anywhere on your partner's body or use them in your hands to determine if they are an appropriate temperature.

The placed stones promote relaxation and grounding with their weight and heaviness. If your partner is prone to anxiety and tension, has a feeling of flying in a lot of different directions, or is fidgety, placing stones has much the same effect as swaddling a baby. There is a certain security and comfort in being held or having pressure resting on one's body.

1. PLACE STONES BENEATH THE BODY

You may choose to have your partner lie on stones and place them on top of his body. Some people are not comfortable lying on stones, in which case it is fine to leave them out. If you do choose to place stones under your partner, have him sit up from a supine position to place them. Place two of your largest, relatively flat, stones on each side of his vertebral column at his waist level and just above, allowing about 1 inch (2.5 cm) between them so that his spine will not be on the stones. Place two of your larger working stones above the large placement stones so that there are three on each side of his lower back (photo A). Place a hand towel over the stones and support his back as he lies back onto them. A pillow under the lower thigh/knee area will take strain off his lower back.

Health Benefits of Hot Stone Massage

- Promotes muscle and fascia lengthening; reduces muscle spasms and cramps
- Alleviates stress, anxiety, and insomnia
- Helps release toxins and oxygenate the tissues
- Improves circulation
- Calms the mind and body; can be very meditative
- Warms cold extremities and is useful for Raynaud's syndrome (a neurovascular condition in which fingers and toes have interrupted circulation) as long as sensation is present
- Balances energy
- Is helpful for menstrual cramps
- Is useful in relief of noninflammatory arthritis pain and fibromyalgia
- Is very grounding and stabilizing
- Can be useful for stimulating reflex points in the feet and hands
- Can relieve pain and congestion in the sinuses when stones are applied to sinus acupressure points on the face

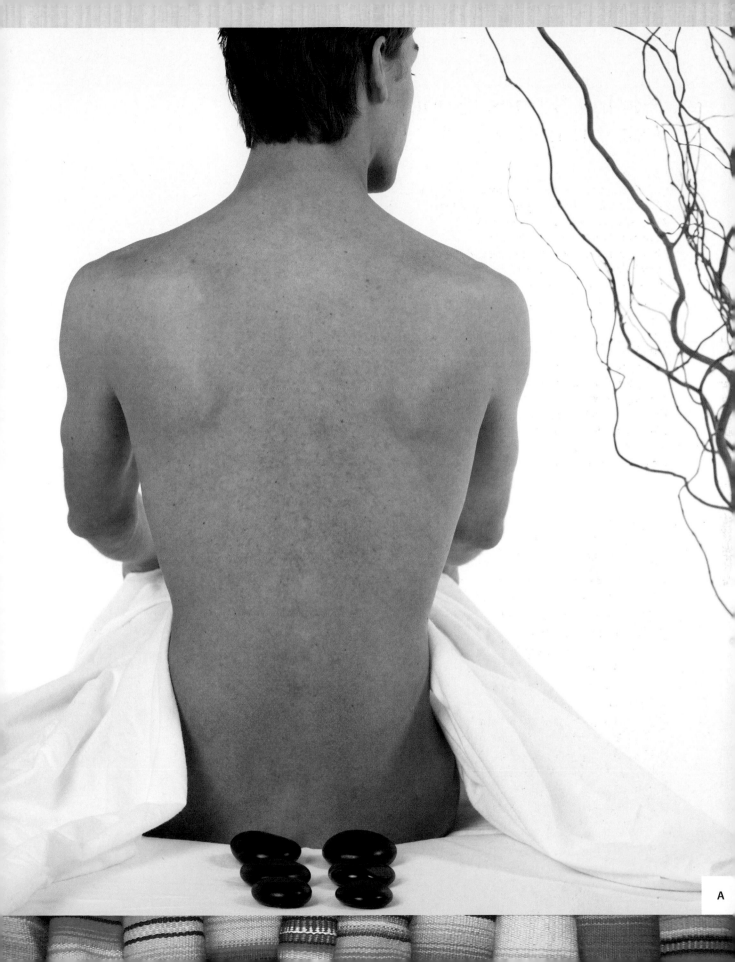

A

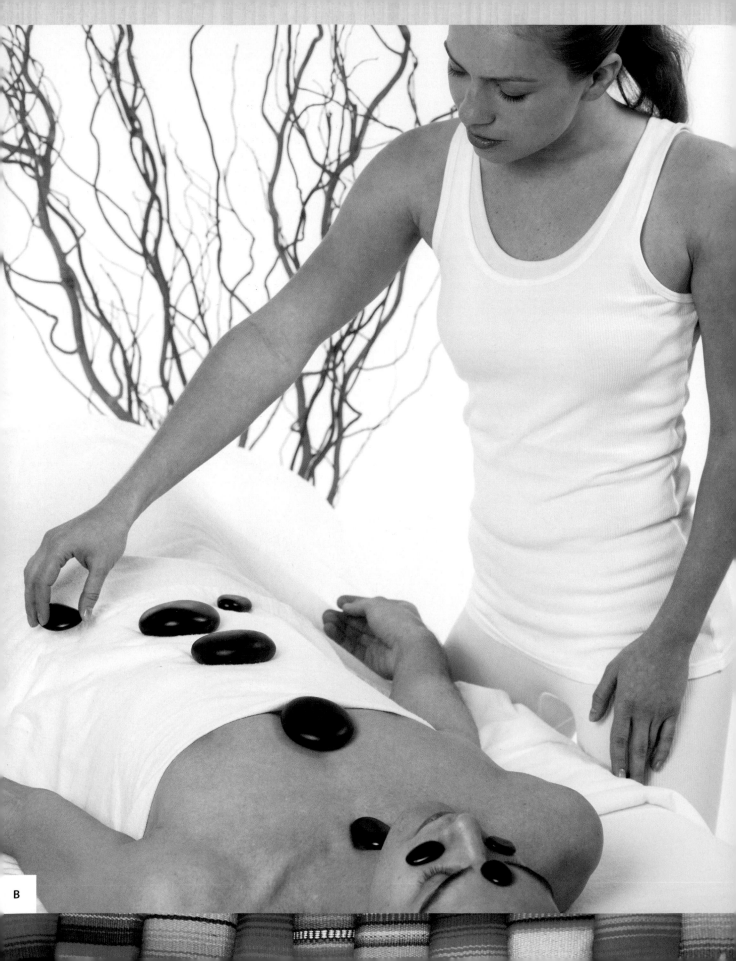

2. PLACE STONES ON THE CHAKRA CENTERS

Starting at your partner's head, place a toe stone on the middle of his forehead, just above his eyebrows on the third eye chakra point (see "Chakra Sequence" in chapter 4). This is an interesting stone placement and it often will interrupt the receiver's train of thought. Frequently, a receiver will stop talking mid-sentence as you replace the forehead stone with a warmed one during a session.

Place two more toe stones on your partner's cheekbones. If you have a rice-filled eye pillow, placing it over his eyes and the stones will help keep the cheekbone stones in place. The next stone to place is the throat chakra stone, which should fit in the hollow above your partner's sternum, at the base of his neck.

You may place the heart chakra stone, a medium-size working stone, on top of the sheet covering your partner's chest, with the top of the sheet folded down over the stone so that it cannot slide toward your partner's throat. Place the solar plexus chakra stone, another medium-size working stone, over the sheet at the base of your partner's sternum, at the top of his abdomen.

Place the sacral chakra stone over the sheet just below your partner's navel. This may be a large placement stone or a medium-size working stone; ask your partner about the weight if you use a large placement stone. Place two small palm-size working stones at each groin; these are about as close as you can come to placement on the root chakra and correspond to the ovaries in women (photo B).

3. PUT STONES IN HANDS AND ON FEET

Place a small to medium-size working stone in each of your partner's hands and take the handkerchief of toe stones to the foot of the table, placing the stones between all of his toes. An optional placement is to put a pair of slightly cooled medium-size working stones on the pillow supporting your partner's knees, just behind his knees; this is a tender area, so it's especially important that the stones not be too hot.

It is important to realize that the small toe stones cool down very rapidly, while the larger stones retain heat for up to ten minutes on top of the body and slightly longer if they are underneath. You may want to replace the toe, throat, and facial stones periodically during a massage session.

You could end the massage at this point after the stones begin to cool or continue the session using stones to perform Swedish massage strokes on your supine partner or turning him over and placing stones on his back.

Moving Hot "Working" Stones (Supine Sequence): Ironing Out the Kinks

Have Replacement Stones Ready to Go

When you retrieve stones from the skillet, consider removing an extra pair to exchange with the ones you first use on your partner's arms. Moving stones over the body pulls the heat out of them fairly quickly. As you work with stones, you will notice that the heat is pulled much faster from the side of the stone you are moving on your partner's body than the side against your palm. You can learn to quickly and unobtrusively flip the stone as you massage to bring the warmer side into contact with your partner's body.

Although much of the time in a hot stone massage you will be applying the stones directly to your partner's skin, for at least half of the massage time you will use your hands directly on him. Start massaging each area of his body with your hands to spread lubricant and to acquaint yourself with the quality and tightness of the tissues. Then use the hot stones as tools to enhance your ability to soften and relax the areas you have determined need them the most. Because you will be handling the stones, your hands will feel hot, and at times your partner may not be able to determine whether it is your heated hand or a stone that is moving over his body.

EXPERIMENT WITH HOLDING A HOT STONE

You can hold a hot stone in different ways when you use it as a working stone. The most superficial stroke with a hot stone, and perhaps the most commonly used, is to place the stone flat in your palm and use it as though your palm is simply thicker and hotter. Effleurage is the easiest technique to use with hot stones, as they fit easily in the palms and you can curl your fingers around them without difficulty. Lifting or spreading strokes are also well suited to stone use. You may push a stone lying flat on the tissues with the heel of your hand, your fingers, or the thumbs and index fingers of both hands. You may turn a stone up on its edge and use the broad edge like a scraper; this move is useful for working more deeply in areas such as the feet, which are accustomed to considerable pressure. You may also use the narrow edge of a stone just lateral to the spine or along the medial edge of a shoulder blade.

Integrating the use of hot stones in a basic massage session (**photo A**) requires practice. Over time, you'll get to know your stones and their cooling rates and energetic properties, which ones fit your hands well, which are stable to place on certain areas of the body, and which are very smooth or have some useful texture. Although the distinction is made here between placement stones and working stones, in practice there is a flow between them. Since the working stones can be hotter than those you place on your partner's body, as a working stone begins to cool down you can place it to capture the remaining heat. Follow your intuition regarding placement of "spent" working stones and remove them as they lose their heat. They will remain noticeably warm for five or ten minutes, depending on their size.

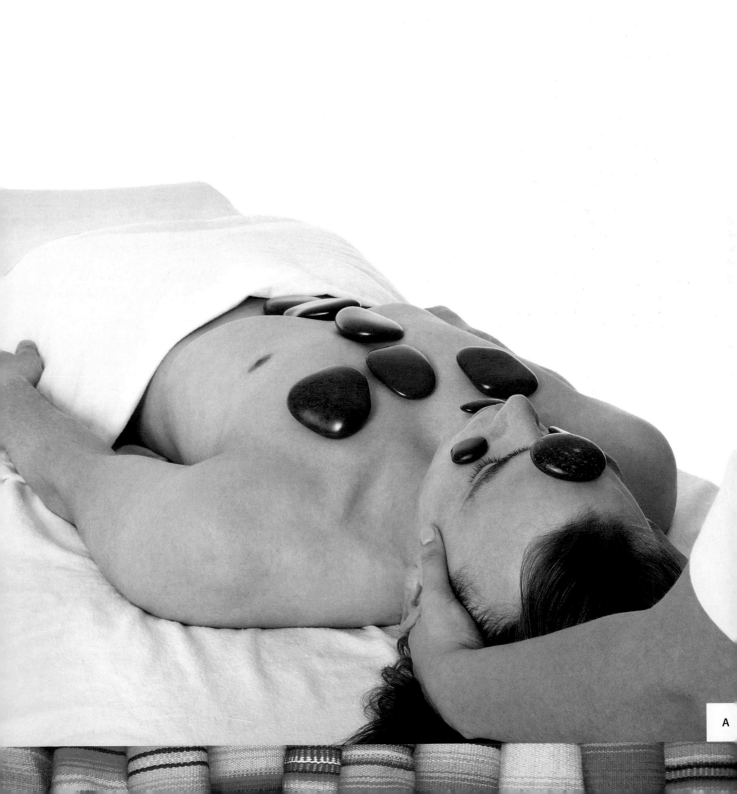

A

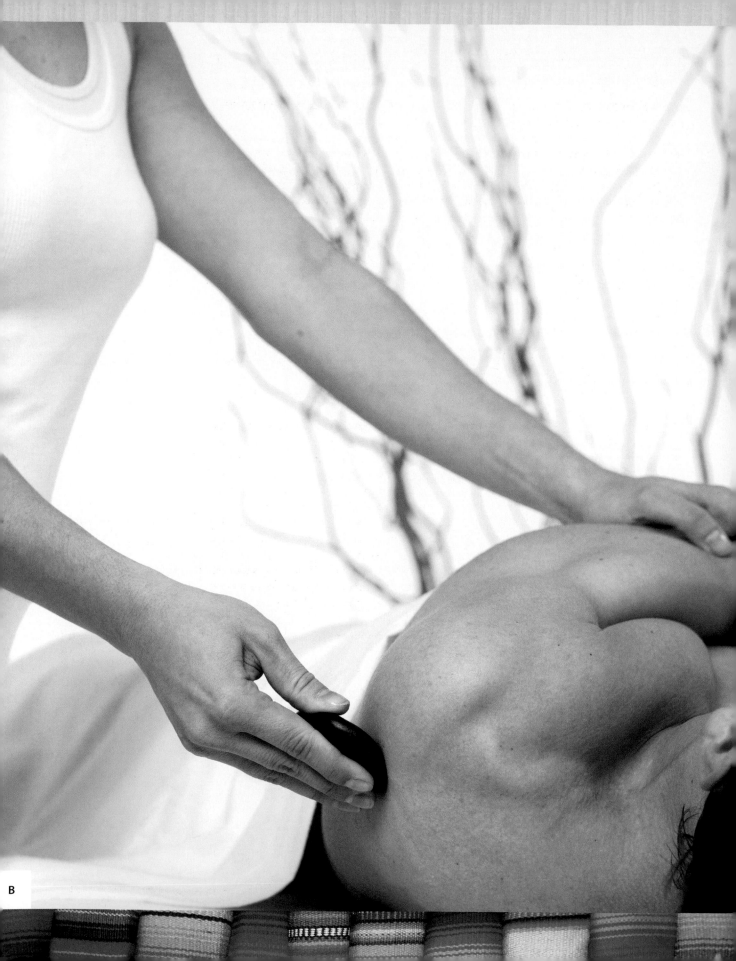

1. BEGIN WITH THE HAND AND ARM

The hand, which is accustomed to temperature changes, is much more forgiving than more sensitive or touchy areas of the body. Remove the stone resting in your partner's hand and use effleurage from his fingertips all the way up and around his shoulder to spread lubricant and to get a sense of tight areas in his hands, arms, and shoulders. After you spread the lubricant, use two small palm stones to effleurage the same area. As you explore your partner's arms and find tight spots and knots, you may want to pick up one of your small working stones and hold it on the tight area for a few breaths, compressing with the heat and weight of the stone to soften and release knots.

2. USE STONES BETWEEN THE SPINE AND SHOULDER BLADE

When you take your partner's arm across his chest and reach under his back to the medial border of his scapula, have a stone in your palm to apply firm friction along the medial edge of his shoulder blade (photo B). This will enhance the upper back stretch you are encouraging by rocking or pressing your partner's elbow away from you and across his chest. The stone will distract and therefore soften the upper back muscles. You may leave the stone between his scapula and spine when you return his arm to the table to continue generating heat for the upper back muscles. Remember to place another stone in your partner's hand after you have finished massaging his arm and hand.

Place Large Stones to Relax the Chest

If you notice that your partner's shoulders are elevated above the massage table rather than resting easily on it, you may want to place a large stone on each side of his chest on his pectoral muscles after you massage them with or without a working stone. Place them within the envelope of the turned-down sheet to assist in holding them in place and maintaining their heat as long as possible. The weight and heat of these large stones on your partner's chest may gradually encourage his shoulders to sink to the table surface, opening his chest and relieving associated upper back discomfort.

3. MASSAGE THE HEAD

Follow the Swedish system for massaging your partner's head and neck. With your palms facing down, bring your thumbs together in the middle of his forehead. Linger there with light pressure for a breath and then perform a few spreading strokes all the way out to where his cheek meets the front of his ear. Bring your fingertips together under his chin and sweep your hands slowly up the side of his face to the top of his head a few times, which works like a face lift. Bring your fingers to the side of his nose and trace below his cheekbones out to the front of his ear.

Bring the backs of your wrists to the table surface so that your fingertips curve upward at the base of your partner's skull (the occipital ridge) and apply circular friction back and forth across the ridge with your hands mirroring each other.

Apply Friction to the Lateral Jaw

If your partner holds tension in his jaw muscles, use the toe stones to relax the muscles that contribute to TMJ (temporomandibular joint) problems and related headaches. Use small stones in both hands and apply circular friction at the angle of his jaw on the lower lateral face to release the jaw. Several short, firm, downward "stripping" strokes on the masseter muscle at the angle of the jaw can lengthen the muscle and reduce tightness from grinding teeth, dental procedures, or stress.

Relieve Sinus Pain with Small Stones

You can ease sinus pain and congestion by applying static pressure with small stones at the sides of your partner's nose at the crease and below the iris of each eye just below the cheekbone (photo C). Another option is to use sweeping strokes with warm or cold stones or alternating a few strokes with a warm stone, followed by a few with a cold one from the lateral nose to the ear just below the cheekbone to address the sinus acupressure points. Use hot or cold stones to apply circular friction on the temples to relieve headache discomfort.

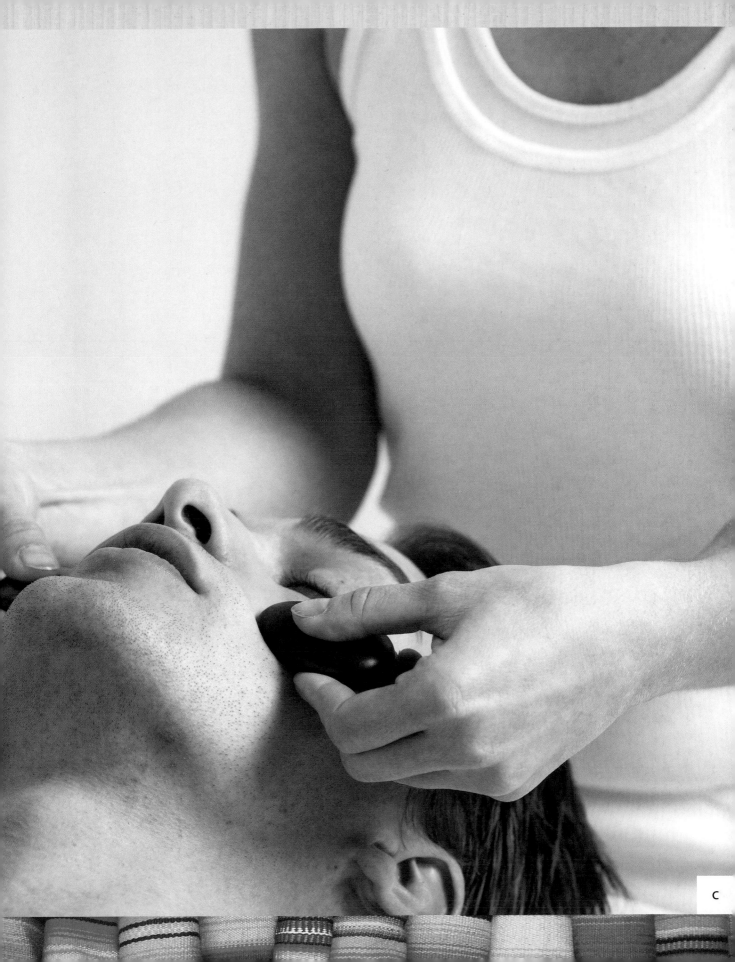

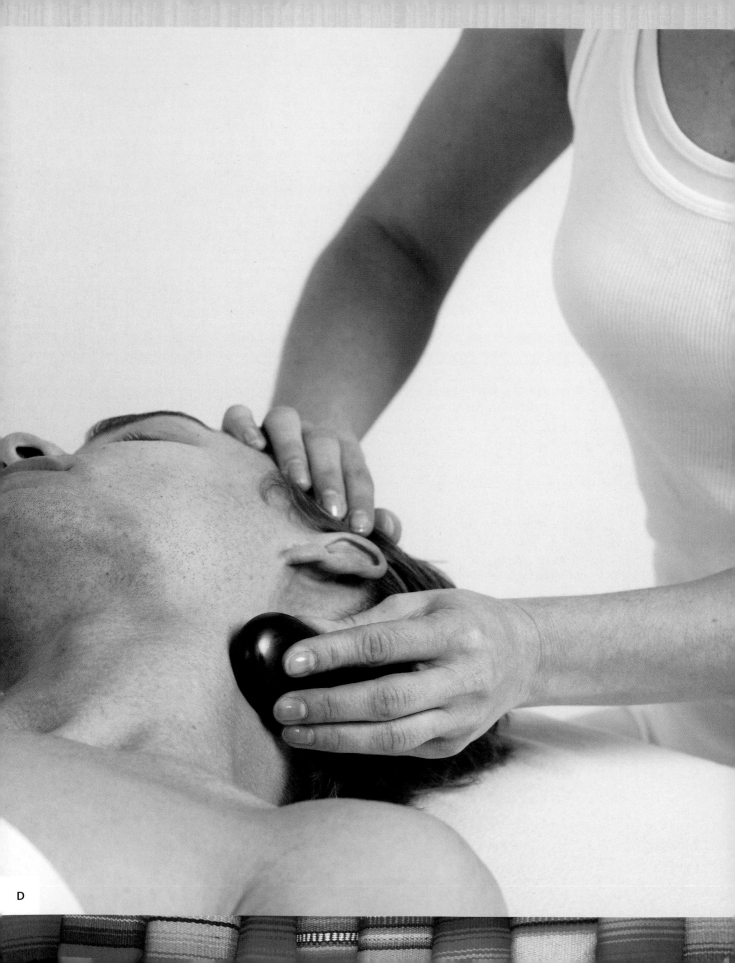

D

4. RELEASE NECK TENSION WITH HOT STONES

Before using stones on your partner's neck, palpate his neck muscles with circular friction at the base of his skull and up and down the muscles on each side of his spine with Swedish massage to acquaint your hands with areas of held tension. Then use two of the smallest working stones to perform between three and five spreading strokes across the occiput and effleurage up and down the back of his neck, staying off the vertebrae.

You may rotate your partner's head to the right and apply long strokes with a hot stone in your right hand from just below his left ear out to almost the tip of his shoulder and back up, repeating the stroke a few times **(photo D)**. Switch the stone for a warmer one before repeating the strokes on the left side of his neck. With his head in a neutral position and a stone in each of your palms, strongly press the stones into the area where his shoulders meet the side of his neck and lean toward his feet. Hold the compression with the stones for at least three breaths.

Hot Stone World History

The therapeutic benefits of a hot stone massage have been known for centuries. Native Americans used hot stones as early as 1,500 BC during sweat lodge ceremonies to detoxify and to enhance their meditative experience, and they assisted laboring women with the application of hot stones. In Europe, hot stones or bricks wrapped in cloth were placed over injured areas for healing and pain relief. Mayans are thought to have performed healing rituals with hot stones 5,000 years ago. In Asian cultures, hot stones that were also pointed were used long before needles in treatments closely related to acupuncture, balancing and channeling energy along the meridian lines to improve the functioning of internal organs. Stones were also used for healing work in Africa, Egypt, and India. The baths of the ancient Roman Empire used applications of heat and cold to stimulate healing, including heated stones.

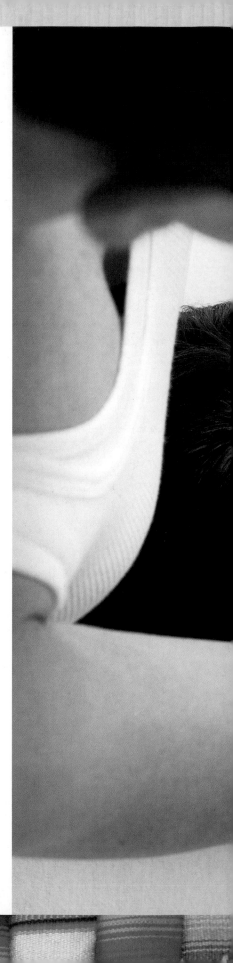

The Magic of Hot Stones

Hot stones have energetic and magnetic properties. They also have very calming, sedative, and meditative qualities. Hot stones feel good to the giver as well as the receiver of massage and can add depth to strokes without more effort.

5. REMOVE STONES TO MASSAGE THE CHEST

After you have moved to the head of the table and massaged your partner's head, neck, and upper shoulders, the large stones that you put on his chest will have transferred their heat and weight. Remove them and use a medium-size working stone in each hand to apply effleurage from the center of his upper chest outward **(photo E)**; then come all the way around his shoulder joints and up the back of his neck a few times. You can add placement stones on his chest again if tightness is still apparent in his pectoral muscles. You may also lean your forearm on one of the chest placement stones for a few breaths to enhance the effect of the stone's weight, but check in and make sure your partner does not experience any numbness or tingling in his arm or hand as you apply the weight.

6. MOVE TO THE LOWER BODY

Moving to the lower body, first remove any stones that may still be between your partner's toes or behind his knees. Spread lubricant on his leg and foot and then use your largest working stones to effleurage his legs and thighs. Apply circular and spreading strokes on his thighs and spreading strokes from his shin down toward the table on his calves. Use a small working stone to apply firm cross-fiber and circular friction all around his knee. Moving the edge of a stone back and forth just below the kneecap (patella) addresses the tendons for all the quadriceps muscles. Bringing your partner's foot onto the table surface with his heel close to his buttocks, begin to lean and rock his leg away as you massage the lateral thigh. Use a hot stone to glide up and down his thigh, sensitively encouraging it to move farther across his opposite leg, while applying effleurage strokes or a series of compressions. This will tend to create length in the posterior pelvis and a feeling of flexibility and space in the hip.

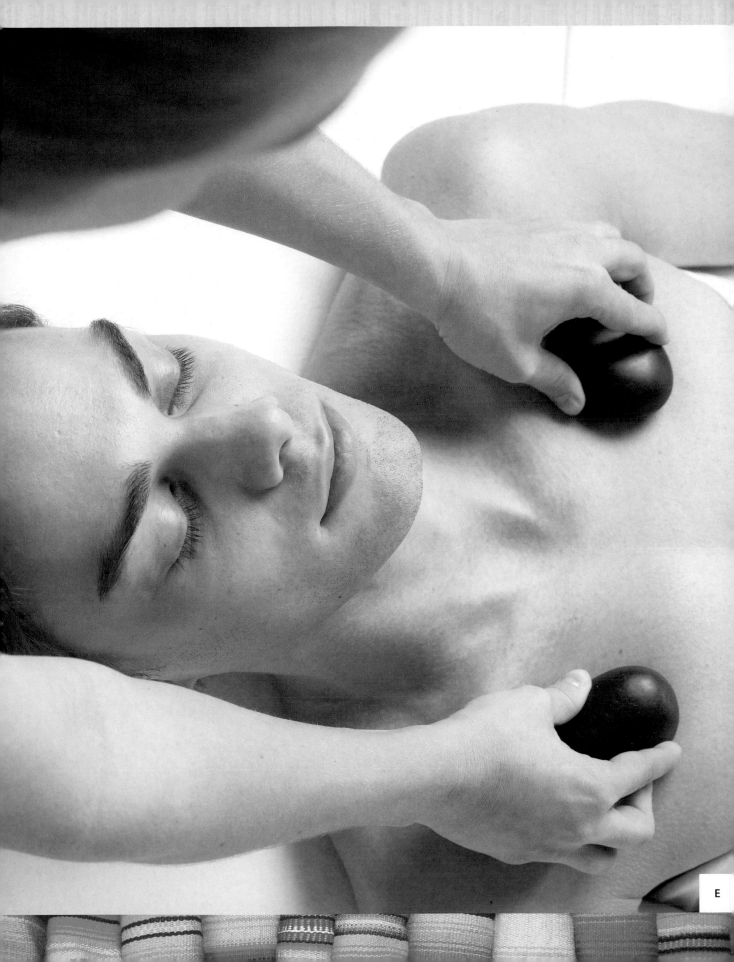

Massage the Hip and Hamstrings with Stones

With your partner's leg leaning away from you with one hand, you can use a stone in the other hand to massage around his hip joint and into the lateral buttock muscles while they are in a stretched position, further opening the hip (photo F). Depending on your partner's flexibility and your relative sizes, you may be able to face the head of the table, kneeling near his hip, and place his foot on your shoulder. You can then lubricate and warm his hamstrings with several effleurage strokes. With a medium-size working stone in each hand you can work both sides of these hamstring muscles by gliding or compressing with the stones as you lean forward to keep his knee moving closer to his chest. This not only begins to address the hamstrings but stretches the lower back as well.

When you release your partner's leg, rotate his knee out to the side and place his foot near his opposite knee, with a pillow or your knee underneath if his leg does not rest easily on the table. Apply effleurage strokes from the medial knee to the groin first with your palms, then with a medium-size working stone, and use circular friction with the stone around the medial knee. You will have addressed the hip joint in the various planes it can move with these stretches, which will lubricate the joint and may improve its range of motion.

7. REMOVE STONES AND TRANSITION TO PRONE SEQUENCE

Remove all the placement stones, remembering those that may be under the sheet or under your partner's body. You can remove stones from under the body in three ways. The first way is to ask your partner to sit up. The second is to reach over his torso and rotate his upper body toward you and push the stones out from under him before you roll him onto his back again. The third way is to get him to roll onto his side away from you and remove the stones before he rolls all the way over to a prone (face-down) position.

Health Benefits of Cold Stone Massage

- Reduces inflammation from strains and sprains
- Stimulates the nervous system
- Provides an analgesic effect by numbing sensations of pain
- Increases muscle tone

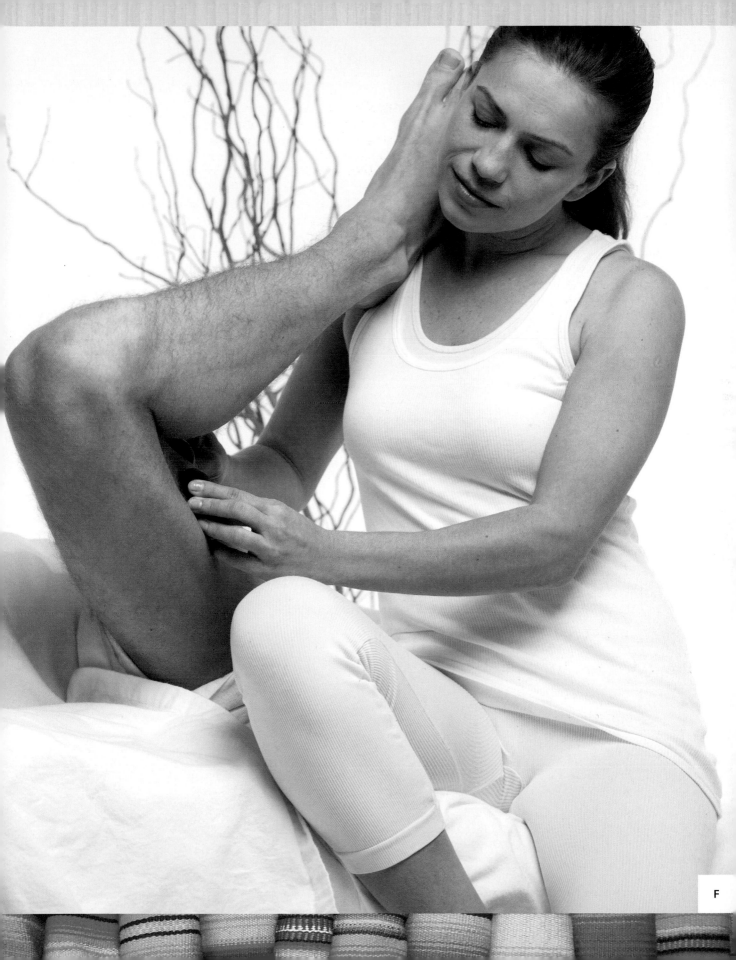

Hot Stone Prone Sequence:
Allowing Heat to Sink In

The weight of large stones placed on the back, combined with the heat that sinks into the back's hard-working postural muscles, melts muscle tension and allows the receiver to release those muscles. There's no need to hold those stones. The use of stones as heated tools on chronically tight hamstrings, gluteal muscles, and back muscles can provide much-needed relief from discomfort due to overuse.

1. PLACE STONES ON BACK

When your partner is in the prone position, place the largest stone on his sacrum. Then place three large stones on each side of his vertebral column—up to a level between his scapulas—and one stone in each of his palms **(photo A)**. Undrape and lubricate one of his legs, from the toes to the hip. Follow by using medium-size stones on the entire backs of his legs. Hold the top of his foot in one hand while you work deeply with a stone on the sole of his foot.

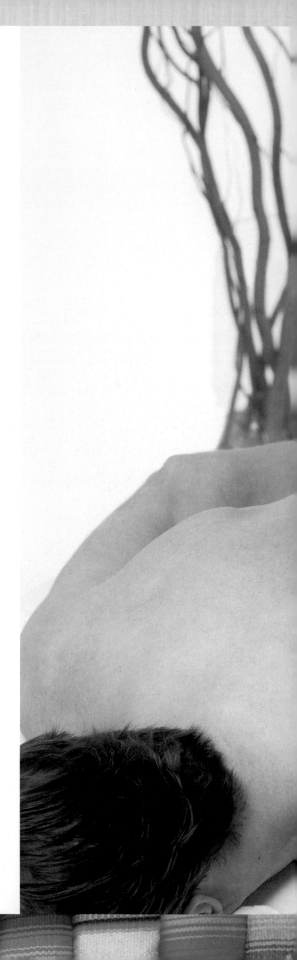

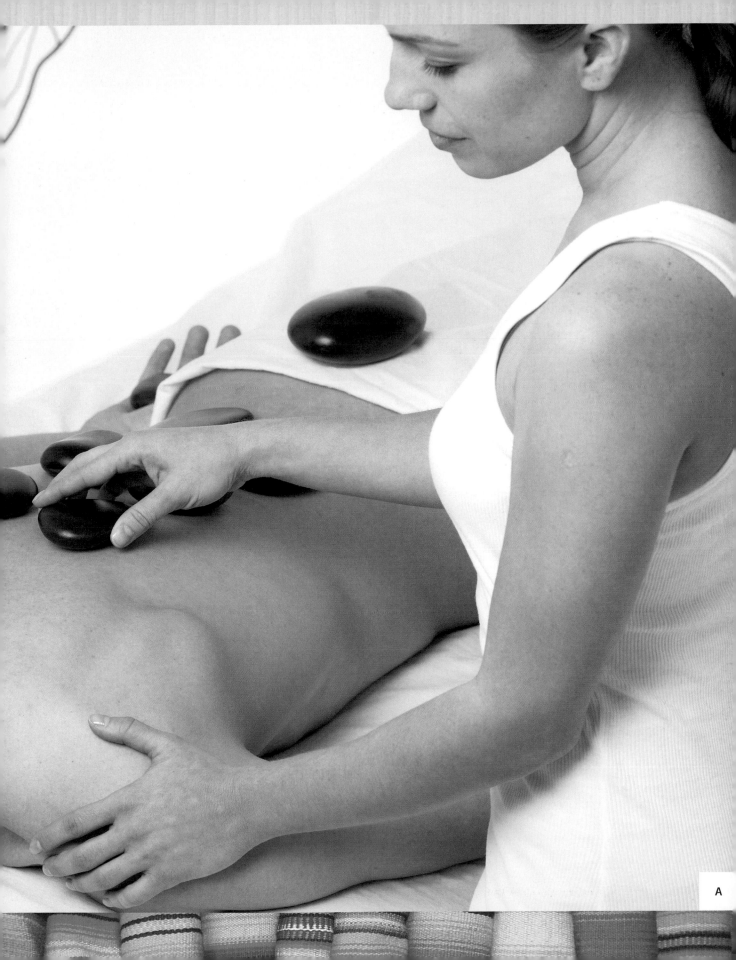

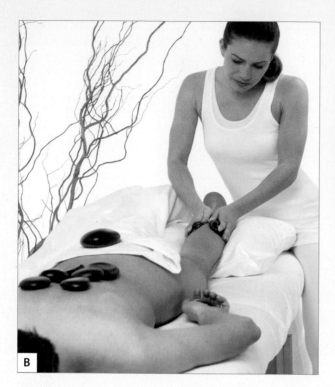

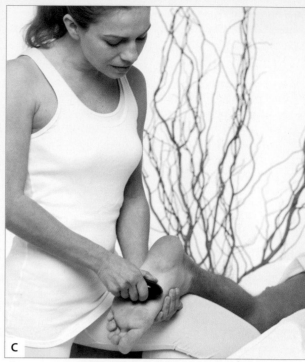

2. MASSAGE THE THIGH, CALF, AND BUTTOCK

Apply several superficial spreading strokes on your partner's thigh and calf muscles and figure eights of effleurage taking in both his leg and thigh (**photo B**). You may either massage the buttock area as an extension of the thigh, performing circular friction around the hip joint and from the sacrum to the hip, or address the gluteal area and hips as an extension of the back. If you place heated stones on the soles of the feet as you complete the massage of the leg, it will feel good to your partner, reminiscent of walking on a hot beach, but the stones tend to slip off onto the table. You may find you have a couple of stones whose shape allows them to remain more securely on the feet. Tucking the sheet around the feet to hold the stones in place can also help secure the stones.

3. SOOTHE THE SOLES WITH HEAT

Cradling your partner's foot in your left hand, use first a small stone held flat in your right hand with moderate pressure between the heel and ball of his foot. You may then turn the stone and work the sole and arch with a scraping motion using the edge of the stone to work more deeply (**photo C**).

4. LENGHTEN BACK MUSCLES WITH STONES

Remove the stones you placed on your partner's back, tapping each with a smaller stone if you like to release energy and create a pleasant vibration under the resting stone. Spread lubricant on his entire back from the head of the table. Use medium-size working stones to apply several long, flowing, gentle effleurage strokes from his shoulders to his hips, back up

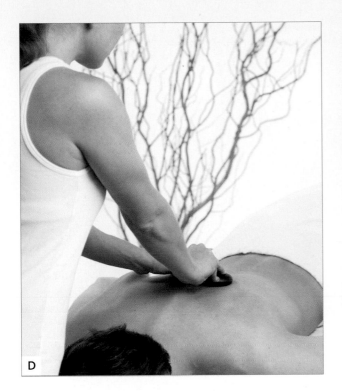

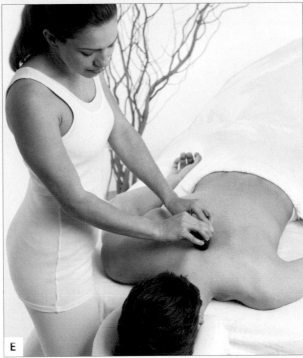

and around his shoulders, and up the sides of his neck **(photo D)**. Stand to one side of the table and perform pushing strokes from the vertebral column to your partner's side, gradually moving toward his shoulders from his waistline **(see photo F, page 72)**. You can use a stone in each hand, or use both of your hands on a larger placement stone for lateral strokes on the back.

5. BROADEN THE UPPER BACK

When you arrive at the area of the scapulas, just move the stone or stones from your partner's spine to the medial edge of the scapula, as going over the edge of the scapula in this direction might be uncomfortable. If your partner's scapulas are close to the spine, you may want to turn the stone on its edge and use it in a

scraper position. Lighten the pressure at the border of the scapula and continue the stroke at an angle up toward the point of your partner's shoulder **(photo E)**. You may use a small stone to apply friction around the borders of the scapula and along the crest of his hip.

6. REPEAT SEQUENCE ON OPPOSITE SIDE OF THE BACK

Undrape the other leg and repeat the entire sequence on the other side.

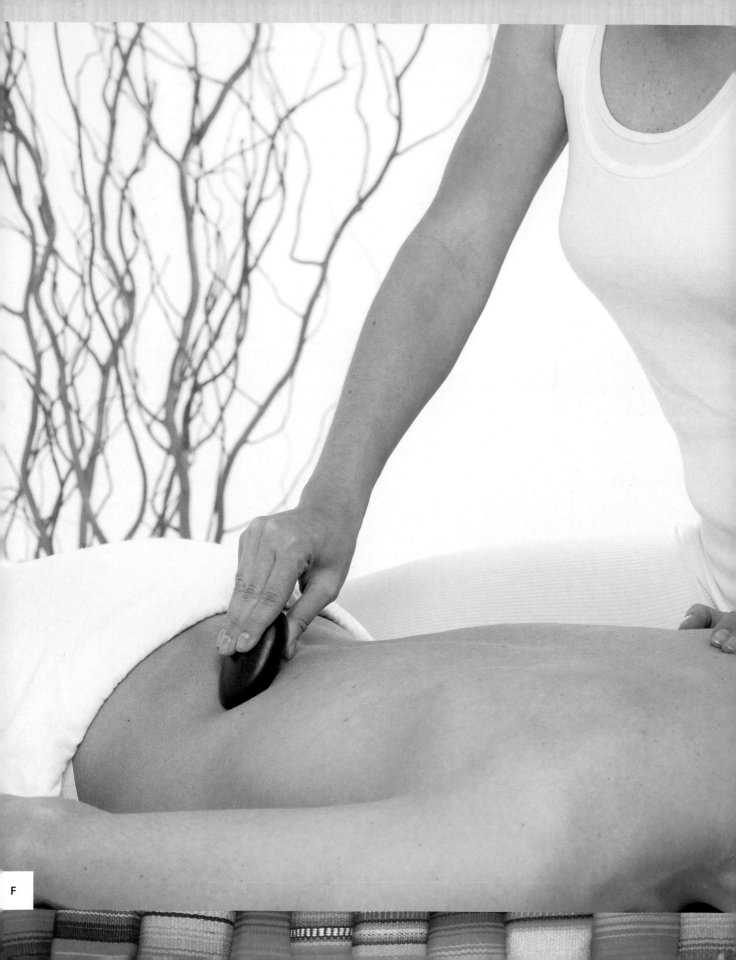

F

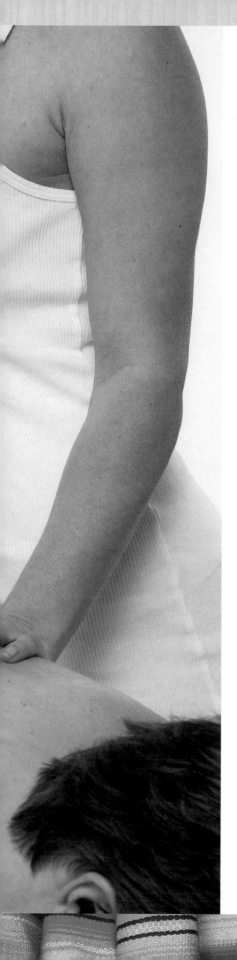

6. FINISH WITH EFFLEURAGE AND A CONTACT HOLD

Return to the head of the table and apply several long effleurage strokes, pressing toward your partner's feet and holding at his upper hips for a couple of breaths to lengthen his spine. Then begin moving the stones in opposite directions along the length of his back, moving your hands quickly in a longitudinal friction stroke and staying well clear of his spine. After one or two more connecting effleurage strokes without stones, place your hands lightly on your partner's back for a closing contact hold, allowing three to five breaths to elapse before breaking contact.

AFTER-SESSION CARE OF STONES

When you have completed a hot stone session, you will need to remove the stones from the water in the electric skillet. If you leave stones in water for extended periods, the same iron content in the stones that gives them some electromagnetic qualities will frequently cause veins of rust to appear on the surface of the stones, disrupting their smoothness and possibly creating rust stains on the handkerchief and hand towel you have in the skillet with them. It is ideal to remove all the stones from the skillet and then wash the skillet and place a clean hand towel inside it. Clean the stones in a sink in hot, soapy water and allow them to dry on a towel before transferring them back into the skillet. Make sure the skillet is unplugged and the cover is dry and back in place to protect your stones from dust and dirt until you are ready to use them again.

Warning! Dizziness May Ensue

At the end of a hot stone massage, your partner may experience lightheadedness or feel dizzy when he stands, especially if he normally has low blood pressure. Encourage him to get up slowly and be there to assist if necessary. It's a good idea for him to drink a big glass of water and remain seated until wooziness passes. Scheduling a hot stone massage before work or strenuous physical activity is not ideal, so try to give your partner a hot stone session when you know he can rest and relax afterward.

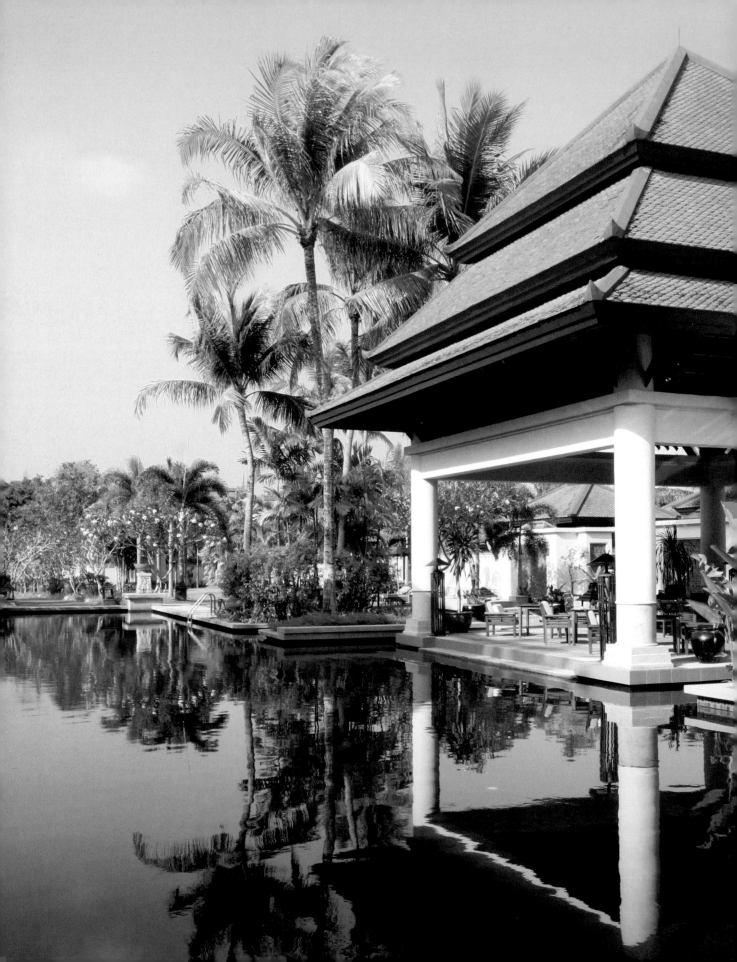

CHAPTER 3

Thai Yoga Massage Integrates Mind, Body, and Spirit

In Thai yoga massage, the receiver is passively placed in a variety of yoga postures on a floor mat. The postures stretch the various energy lines—or sen lines—of the body. The sen lines are also stimulated by palming and thumbing strokes administered by the person giving the massage.

Most of us spend a lot of time in front of computers, driving, or in other stationary positions. Thai massage eases associated stiffness through assisted yoga stretches to make muscles more pliable. Creating space in the body through movement promotes improved blood and lymph circulation. This provides enhanced cellular health and nutrition, and benefits the skin and internal organs, as well as digestion, elimination, and respiration.

Basic Movements in Thai Yoga Massage

Closed kneeling posture

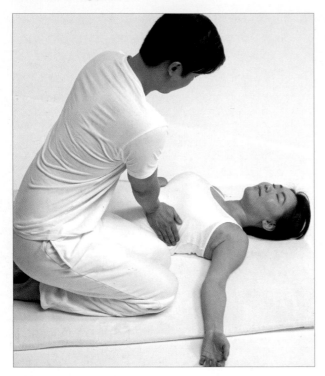

Open kneeling posture

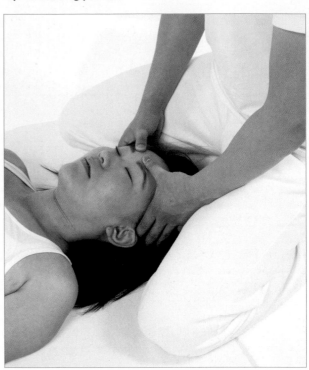

The breath is key in Thai massage; it is the bridge for connecting with your partner. Your breath should be synchronized with your movements and with your partner's breath. Recognize that when you palm your partner's back, you are inducing her to exhale, so make sure you time your compressions with her rate of respiration.

You will use **closed kneeling** and open **kneeling postures**, with the hips toward the heels and knees either together or apart; **kneeling warrior**, with one foot forward on the floor and the knee of the other leg grounded; and standing warrior, with one leg and foot forward with the knee flexed, and the other far back with the knee extended.

Kneeling warrior (front view)

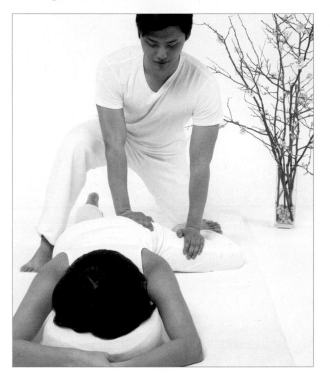

Open kneeling posture (with support)

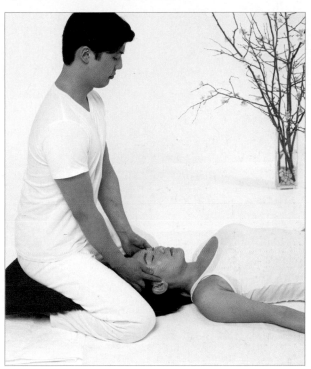

The kneeling stances can be difficult if your legs are inflexible. If this is the case, you can place an extra pillow under your thighs or between your legs and thighs, to reduce strain on your knees (see photo above).

Giving a Thai session requires some strength and agility. Practice will improve your fluidity and grace of movement as well as ease of breath and joint flexibility. Both the giver and the receiver of Thai massage reap many of the same benefits, including improved range of motion, balance, and flexibility, as the moves draw from tai chi, yoga, and chi kung.

Rock for Depth, Not Pressure

The Forward Rock

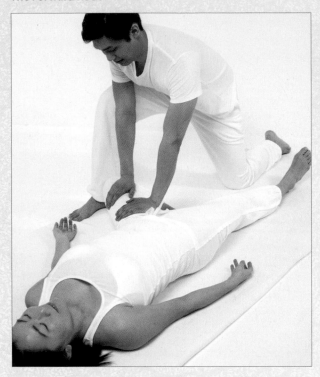

The Side Rock

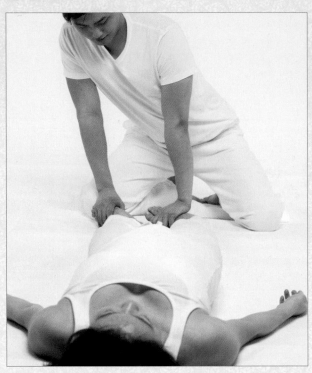

There is a difference between depth and pressure. Many techniques that use stretching or energy manipulation can have a very deep and therapeutic effect without the application of a lot of pressure. Massaging with finesse rather than force is generally preferable, for both the giver and the receiver.

The depth achieved in Thai yoga massage comes mechanically from the sensitive gradual stretching of the muscles and energetically from stimulating points along the sen lines, which form the energetic anatomy of the body. Stretching will be felt more deeply by those who are less flexible; palming and thumbing effects are not dependent on the amount of pressure exerted, but on sinking in slowly with the breath, which will have a much deeper effect than entering the tissue quickly and causing muscles to "guard" and push back.

Palming

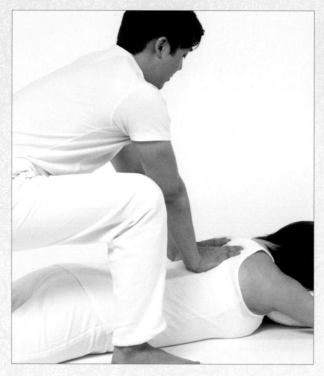

Thumbing

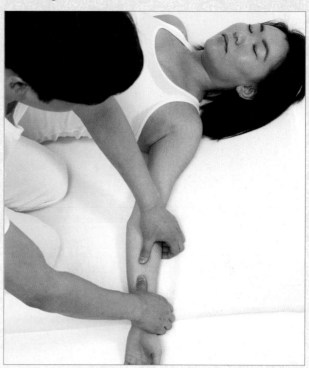

Some standard movements are related to the rhythmic, dance like quality of Thai yoga massage:

The Forward Rock—a rocking-chair type of movement that applies pressure through both palms as they transmit the forward movement of your torso

The Side Rock—a lateral rocking movement in which you apply pressure with the hand on the side of the body toward which you are rocking

Palming—rocking the weight of your body onto your relaxed, soft palm, with your wrist in a neutral position, sinking in and avoiding abrupt pressure

Thumbing—rocking the weight of your body onto the pad of your thumb, with the thumb joint neutral

Prepare the Mat and Your Mind

Both you and your partner should be dressed in loose, comfortable clothing that allows you to move freely. Cotton clothing is a good choice. Avoid fabrics that are too slick to maintain your secure hold on a limb. Traditionally, Thai massage is done with bare feet, but you may want to try yoga socks that have rubber dots to minimize slipping. Your partner may wear socks or have bare feet. Remember that a relaxed person's temperature may drop, so have a blanket available.

In addition to a firm mat, have handy at least two pillows, or a pillow and a kneeling pad. A face cradle or rolled towel is also useful. You can play music to enhance the experience, or you may work in meditative silence. Honor the time, the space, and your partner with mindful preparation.

A MEDITATIVE PRACTICE

To begin a Thai massage session, you should enter a clear centered and meditative state. Create a quiet, calm environment, letting go of outside concerns. Take the time to prepare physically by stretching and moving in sync with your breath. Perform a seated or walking meditation to clear your mind. Doing so will awaken your life force energy known as chi or prana, enabling you to attune with the receiver's energy more easily. Open your heart and set your intention for a sacred healing encounter.

Thai massage has at its core the same fundamental benefits of meditation and other mind/body practices. Intense focus and coordinated breath clears the mind, quieting it and promoting serenity for both giver and receiver. The conscious movement of the postures is a rhythmic, connected, and fluid dance that promotes self-healing. The connection between the giver and receiver is facilitated through a shared breathing pattern; the rhythmic rocking dance of the postures; and metta, or loving kindness which creates harmony between the giver and receiver.

SOFTEN JOINTS AND ROCK THREE TIMES

Be sure to extend your arms and wrists with softness in the joints, so they transmit the rocking movements of your body. Do not rely on tiring contractions of your arm, hand, and shoulder muscles, which can cause repetitive strain injuries. Sink in slowly and avoid abrupt moves, which can be jarring and painful. Hand and arm positions and actions are simple and maintain wrists in a relatively neutral position, without strongly flexing or extending the joints.

Each action is performed about three times, although when you are thumbing and palming sen lines, the pattern is to palm, then thumb, then palm again, rather than perform three repetitions of each action. If your partner has particular areas of tightness or discomfort, spend more time and focus on those areas, until you feel the tissues softening. By coordinating your breath with your rocking movements and remaining relaxed and focused, your

Custom-Design Your Routine

Performing all the sequences in this chapter would take at least ninety minutes; in the interest of time, you may certainly pick and choose from the three seated, three supine, and one side-lying sequence detailed here. The sequences are designed to facilitate flowing transitions, which make Thai massage relaxing to receive. Although the sequences are meant to be flowing and connected, you may pause between postures to give your partner an opportunity to integrate what you've been doing. If certain postures or transitions do not work well for you, adjust them to fit your needs. This is probably why such a huge variety of Thai moves have developed over the centuries!

Seated Sequence One:
Stretch Neck and Upper Shoulder Muscles

The seated sequence in Thai yoga massage offers the giver the mechanical advantage of being able to lean into the upper shoulders, and it stretches the back, neck, and shoulders, making use of gravity to enhance the effects of the strokes.

1. BE GROUNDED WITH DEEP BREATHING

Start by having your partner sit cross-legged, or with legs extended if that is more comfortable, in an erect, relaxed posture. Stand behind her with your palms together in front of your heart. Take a few long breaths to make sure you are centered in your heart and mind and are grounded in your body. Your deep breathing will remind your partner to breathe deeply as well.

2. LUNGE AND LEAN, PALMING SHOULDERS

Place your hands on your partner's shoulders and bring the lateral edge of one foot forward so that it is slightly beneath her tailbone, with your leg supporting her back (**photo A**). This pigeon-toed placement ensures that the muscle of your lower leg, rather than your shin, supports her back. Her spine should be erect, neither listing forward nor slumping. Your other leg should be extended well behind you; the farther back it is and the more weight you have in that foot, the more stable your stance.

Sink your weight into her upper shoulder muscles, exhaling as you sink in and inhaling as you decrease the pressure. Alternate your hand positions from fingers forward and out to the side, gradually leaning more heavily. Keep your hands close to where her neck meets her shoulders and repeat the palming until you feel that her shoulders have relaxed and softened.

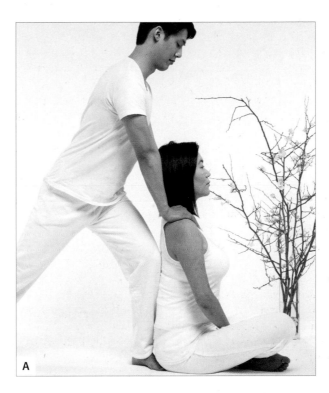

A

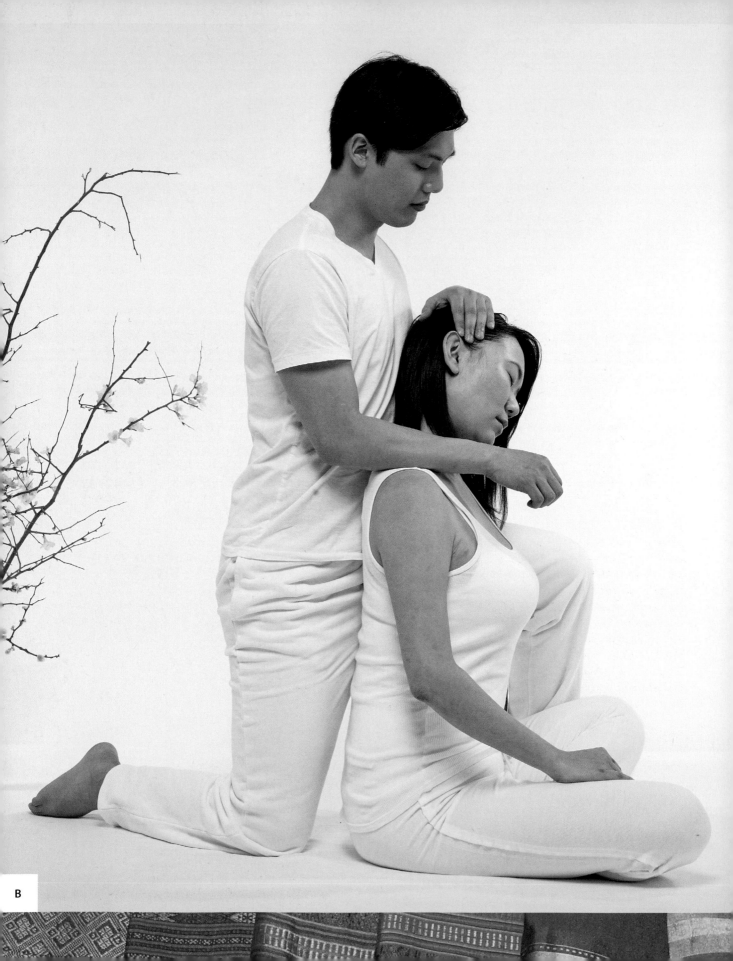

Palm down

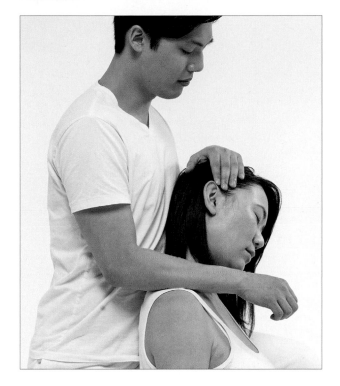

Palm up

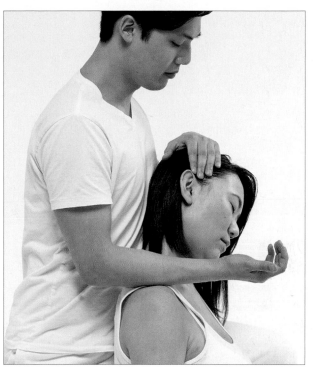

3. ROLLING PIN ALONG THE SHOULDER

Keeping your hands in place to support your partner, drop your right knee to the mat and bring your left foot forward. Place her left arm across your thigh, noticing whether you need to adjust your foot placement to keep her shoulders level **(photo B)**. Gently and slowly flex her neck toward her left shoulder and use just the weight of your left hand to create a gentle lateral stretch as you roll your right forearm from her neck to her shoulder, rolling her arm from **palm down** to **palm up** while you sensitively lean weight into her shoulder. Both the palming and the rolling of the shoulders in this way helps release common tension and discomfort in the upper trapezius muscles. You will feel her shoulders lower as the muscles relax.

4. ROTATE THE ARM AROUND

Grasp your partner's right elbow and bring her arm up, holding her right elbow in your right hand and her right hand in your left hand, and slowly rotate her shoulder so that it sweeps back over her head and forward several times, keeping her forearm level with the floor and her upper arm close to her head (photo C). Be especially cautious if your partner has a history of shoulder dislocations. Your torso will support her back. Be careful to honor any restrictions, keeping the rotation comfortable and safe.

Place her right hand behind her neck and bring her right elbow closer to her head with your left hand as you use your entire right palm to gently squeeze up and down her arm. These compressions increased range of motion in the triceps and shoulder. Check to make sure your partner's shoulders are above her hips. Perform a few more rotations; then place her arm back in her lap. Reverse your leg position while holding her shoulders and repeat the sequence on her left arm and shoulder.

5. KNEAD THE SHOULDER MUSCLES

Again supporting your partner with your hands on her shoulders, sink down into an open kneeling position. Her back should be against your chest, which provides nice body heat as you lift and squeeze her upper shoulder muscles, firmly kneading from close to her neck out to her upper arms. Most people hold considerable tension in this area, so spend extra time on your partner's shoulders, further relaxing the upper trapezius muscles, which tighten from stress; continue until you feel the muscles soften.

History of Thai Yoga Massage

Traditionally, Buddhist monks provided massage as part of their spiritual practice to all suffering people who visited them at temples. A ancient form of healing touch in Northern Thailand, called Nuad Bo-Rarn, which focuses on gently stretching the receiver, is sometimes called the lazy person's yoga. The Southern style of Thai massage, or Wat Po, uses heavier pressure on key energy points. Kam Thye Chow, a respected Canadian teacher, has popularized Thai yoga massage in North America, incorporating conservative moves from each school. He wisely recognized that Western culture is inclined toward personal injury lawsuits, so Thai yoga massage employs gentler, less aggressive stretches than some traditional techniques.

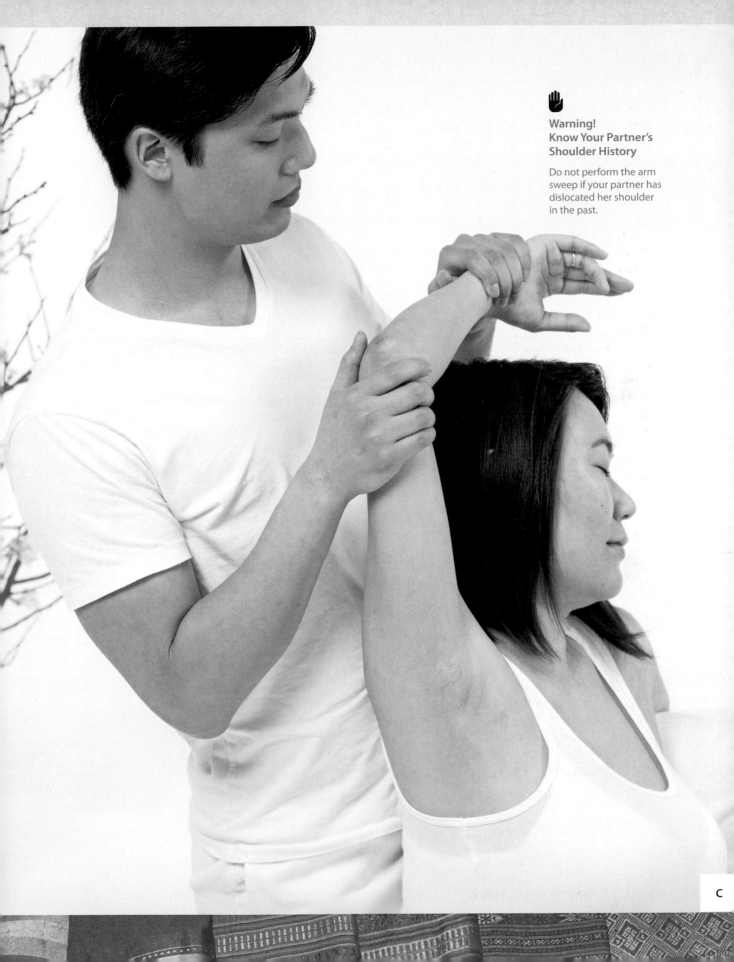

C

Seated Sequence Two: Chest Opening

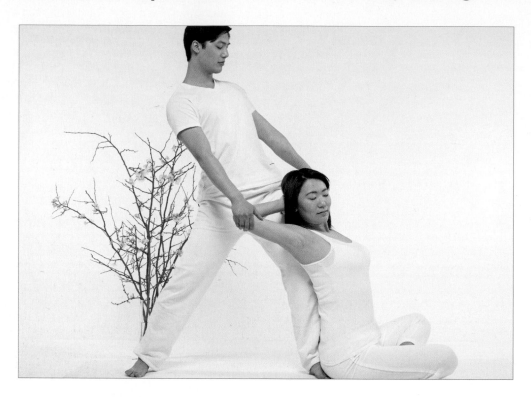

This posture provides a stretch that almost everyone needs: opening the chest—the heart center—with gentle side-to-side movements that help lengthen the pectoral muscles.

1. LIFT THE ELBOWS

Hold your partner's torso upright with your hands on her shoulders while you return to the position you first used, supporting her back with your leg, foot turned medially, but allowing her to lean back by adjusting the position of your leg away from ninety degrees. Reach down and bring her arms up, grasping her elbows. Ask her to lace her fingers behind her neck, and place a hand on each elbow, sensitively pulling one elbow, then the other, up and back toward you, then both elbows at once. This position will open your partner's chest, stretching the pectoral muscles and improving posture, and may reduce referred pain in the arm and hand. Stop if she feels any numbness or tingling in her arms or hands.

Seated Sequence Three: Enhance Back Flexibility

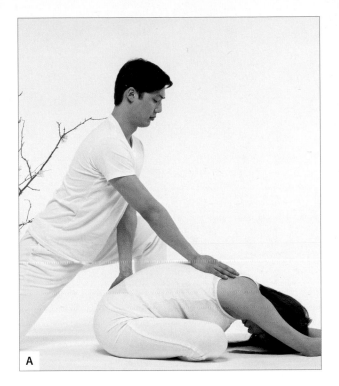

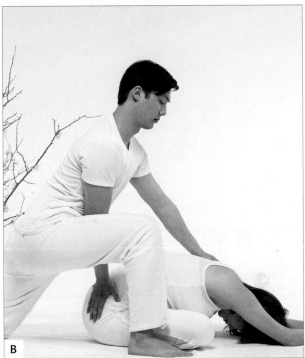

Placing your partner's back in a forward bend stretch while performing compressions and tapotement gradually releases tight postural muscles in the back, passively lengthening them like a relaxing yoga practice.

1. LIFT AND LEAN FORWARD

Lift your partner's hands over her head and lean her forward, with her arms outstretched in front of her and her hands and forearms on the mat. If she lacks flexibility in the forward bend position, have a pillow or two in her lap for support before you lean her forward. Come into a kneeling warrior position behind her and palm the sen lines up each side of her spine, pressing firmly and using your weight on both palms simultaneously as you move from her low back to her shoulders and back (**photo A**). Palm slowly, as you will be inducing her exhalations, as well as coordinating movements with your breath.

As you perform the sequence, your and your partner's breathing rates should gradually slow down. You may also diagonally stretch your partner by palming with one hand on her hip and the other on the opposite shoulder (**photo B**). Palming in the prayer pose will gradually loosen the lower back muscles, increasing flexibility and reducing low back discomfort.

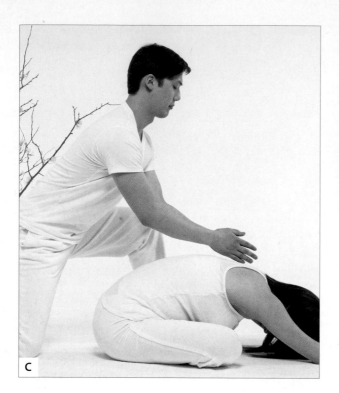

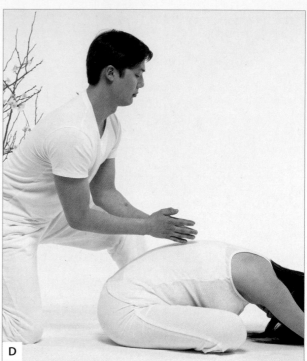

2. HACKING TAPOTEMENT

After palming the sen lines on your partner's back, place your palms loosely together and perform hacking tapotement strokes up and down her back, staying to either side of her spine, stimulating circulation **(photos C, D, and E)**. Assist her back up to a sitting posture then into a reclining, or supine, position, then move to her side. Support her neck as you bring her head and torso to the mat. Extend her legs and make a sweeping stroke or two down each leg to express metta, and to smooth down the pant legs.

Spread Loving Kindness

An expression of metta, or loving kindness, is to sweep your hands lightly at natural breaks in the sequence over the area you've just massaged.

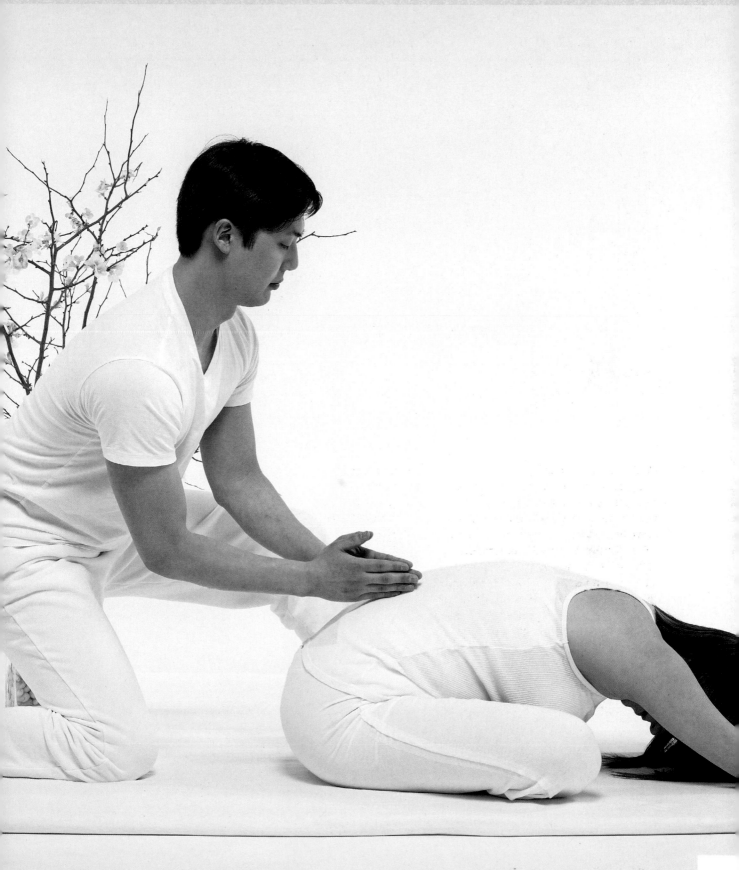

Supine Sequence One: Restore Ankle Flexibility and Reduce Knee and Hip Discomfort

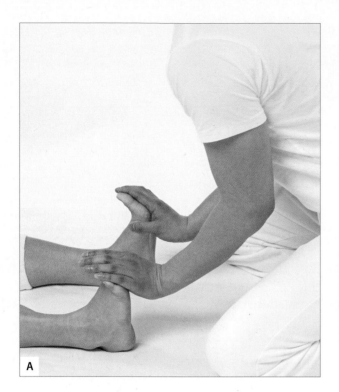

A

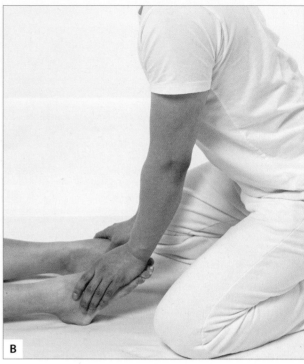

B

This sequence may help restore flexibility to the ankles and result in a more natural stride, or reduce knee and hip pain.

1. PRESS AND ROCK THE FEET

Place a pillow under your partner's head before you move to her feet and assume the open kneeling position to begin the foot and leg sequence. Place both of your hands on her feet and hold for a few breaths before pressing your palms firmly into the arches of her feet a few times, rocking forward with each compression **(photo A)**. Her toes should be pointed out to the sides. Press the soles of both of her feet; then, as you rock back, firmly press the tops of her feet down toward the mat **(photo B)**.

Next, alternately fold each foot medially as you perform the side rock (see "Rock for Depth, Not Pressure" earlier in chapter), gradually moving her feet closer together as you make windshield-wiper movements, and finally folding one foot over the other; then repeat on the opposite side. Many people have tightness in their ankles, which affects the knees and hips as well.

2. THUMB THE SEN LINES OF THE FEET

Starting on the medial sole of your partner's foot at the front of her heel, thumb each sen line on her sole all the way to the tips of her toes **(see illustration)**. Then, hold each side of her foot firmly in your hands and pull one side and then the other a few times, rocking from side to side as you pull. Sweep her lower legs.

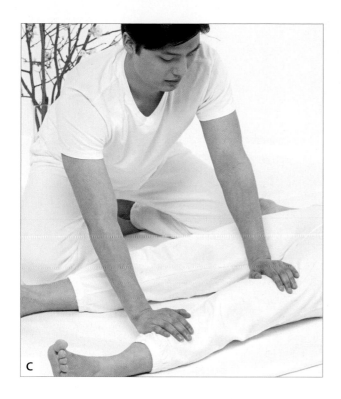

C

Reverse the Energy Flow

Starting a Thai massage at the feet stimulates the flow of energy upward, countering the effects of gravity and encouraging blood and energy that tend to descend through the body to ascend. This creates a balancing effect and energizes the body as a whole.

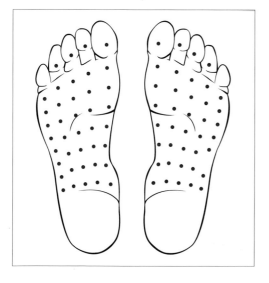

Move forward and to your left so that her foot is between your knees, and thumb the dorsal sen lines on her foot, starting at the ankle and moving to the toes.

3. PALM FROM THE ANKLE TO THE GROIN

Move to your partner's left side, sitting in the open kneeling position by her left leg. Palm from ankle to groin on her far (left) leg, alternating hands, using the side rock (photo C); repeat the same pattern, thumbing the medial sen lines shown in the illustration. Thumbing and palming the area helps to create length in the tendons as well as balances energy along the sen lines, and may reduce muscle imbalances, knee strain, and pain. may reduce muscle imbalances, knee strain, and pain.

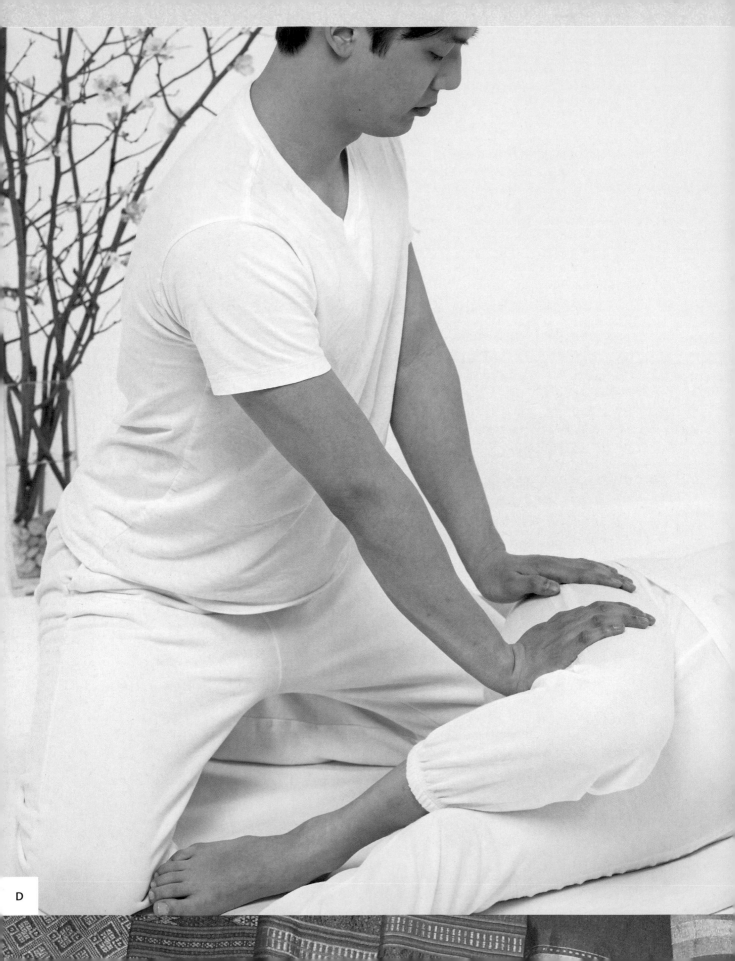

4. STRETCH THE HIP ACROSS THE LEG

Bring your partner's left knee to an upright position with her foot flat on the mat close to her hip, and position yourself in an open kneeling position by her left hip while supporting her upright knee. Begin to rock her hip away from you as you use alternating hands to palm the lateral sen line on her leg, gradually encouraging the leg to move farther over her right leg, but not allowing it much return so that it continues to stretch farther away from you on forward rocks **(photo D)**. This opens the back of the hip area, and is especially helpful for those whose legs turn out strongly when they are lying supine, or who have hip pain that radiates down the lateral legs.

5. PALM THE SEN LINES ON THE THIGH

Move into the kneeling warrior position with your left foot forward and your right knee between your partner's legs. Place her right foot against your abdomen, groin, or shoulder and rock forward, using your palms or the backs of your fingers to palm the medial and lateral sen lines on her posterior thigh from hip to knee **(photo E)**. As you palm up and down the flexed thigh, gradually rock forward a little further with each two-handed palming until her thigh is closer to her chest. This posture passively stretches your partner's lower back, reducing discomfort and helping to create length in the erector spinae muscles.

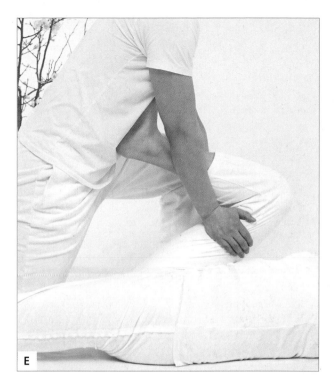

E

Warning—the Back of the Knee Is Delicate!

When palming the back of the thigh and shin, avoid the space directly behind the knee, where there are vulnerable nerves and blood vessels.

Supine Sequence Two: Lengthen Back Muscles, Open Hips, and Loosen Hamstrings

These postures lengthen the back muscles and open the hips, to create a feeling of openness and space in the back, hips, and pelvis. These postures also loosen tight hamstrings.

1. LIFT LEGS AND LEAN BACK TO WIGGLE HIPS

Slowly return your partner to a supine position on the mat. Grasp her heels and lean your weight back as you lift her legs to forty-five degrees or about the level of your waist. Leaning back, move her legs from side to side to wiggle her hips on the mat, then bring her feet up until you feel an end point, asking her to press the backs of her knees toward you. Perform three repetitions, moving her hips and lifting her legs, gradually bringing her legs no more than ninety degrees from the floor. Never force the stretch, but rather encourage the hamstrings to find full extension.

2. FLEX KNEES AND ROCK THE SACROILIAC JOINT

Flex your knees and hips, keeping your knees directly over your partner's hips and placing your toes under the sacroiliac joint on each side by turning your feet into a slightly pigeon-toed position (photo A). Perform a very small side rock, pressing down on her flexed knees. Feel the tiny rocking pressure on your dorsal feet as the movement addresses the pelvis. The sacroiliac joint does not have a large range of movement, and this move helps to prevent it from becoming rigid. Extend your partner's legs and wiggle her hips again before you return her legs to the mat; then sweep her legs.

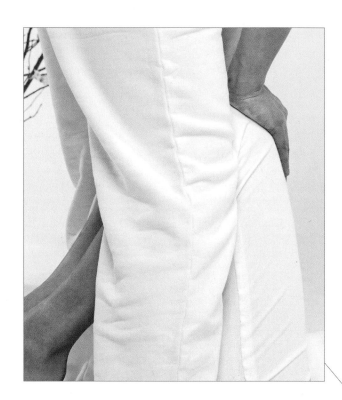

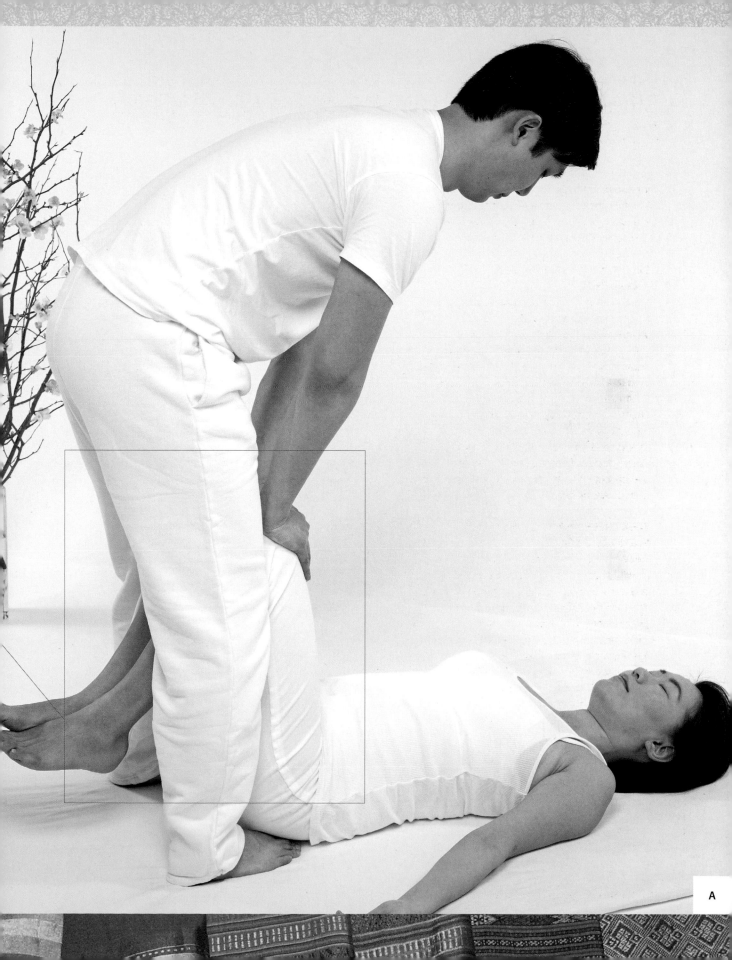

Side-Lying Sequence: Loosening Arm and Shoulder

Assisted twists and shoulder rotations open the body and release muscles in directions we generally don't perform in our activities of daily living.

1. ROLL ONTO THE SIDE AND PALM ARM

Place your partner's arm along the left side of her body, and using one of your hands on her knee (like a lever) and your other hand over hers on her hip, roll her onto her side. Her left knee should remain in a flexed position in front of her extended right leg. Move the pillow if necessary to support her head and neck. Palm and thumb along her arm from wrist to shoulder (photo A).

2. SHOULDER ROTATIONS

With your knees together and your left hip and thigh supporting your partner's back, bring your left hand under her left shoulder and rotate it in circles, moving toward her ear, back, and down, slowly and consciously feeling for the end points in the shoulder's range of motion. These rotations loosen and create ease in all the muscles of the shoulder girdle, including the pectoralis muscles and the lateral neck muscles, which shorten when we routinely have a forward head position to read, or hold a phone to our shoulder. Rotations can ease persistent neck, shoulder, and upper chest discomfort, as well as referred pain down the arm.

Benefits of Thai Massage

- Improves circulation and lowers blood pressure
- Increases joint and muscle flexibility and mobility
- Improves posture and alignment
- Prepares muscles for performance and reduces injuries
- Eases muscle and joint pain
- May deepen respiration
- Boosts the immune system
- Reduces stress and anxiety and improves sleep quality

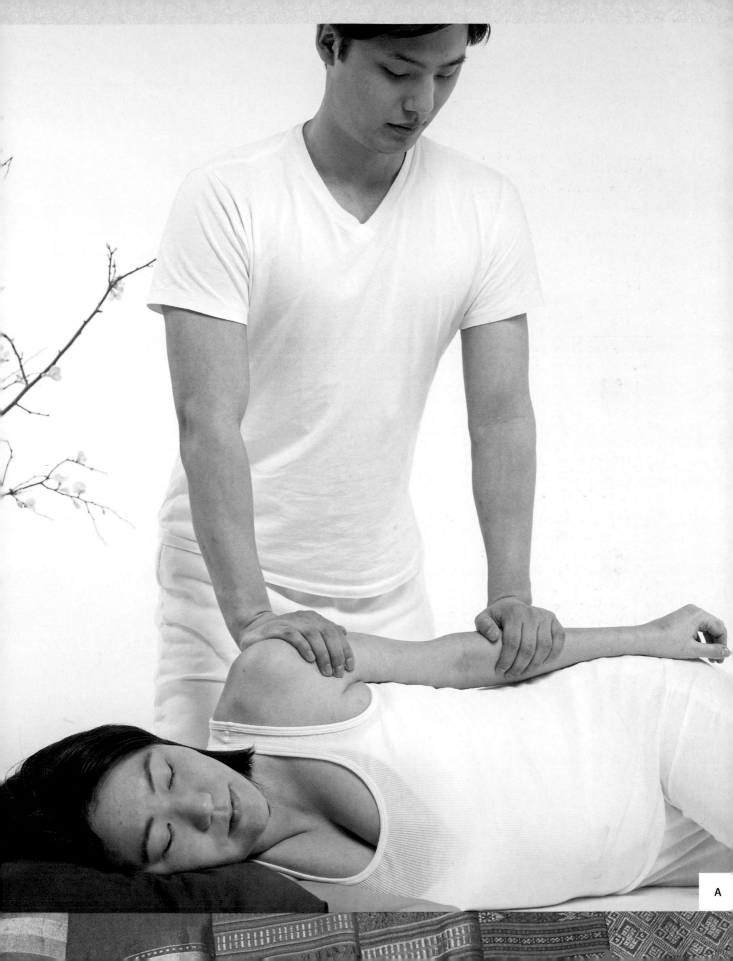

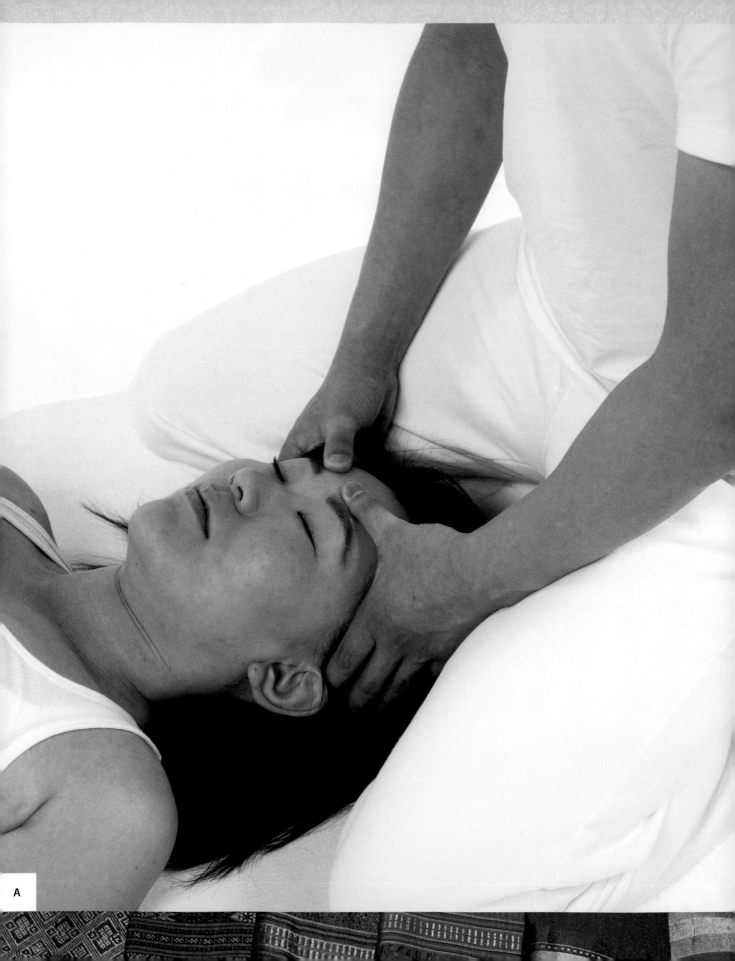

Supine Sequence: Relaxing the Upper Body

1. MASSAGE THE FACE

With your partner lying face up, sit in an open kneeling position or a simple cross-legged position at her head. Thumb her forehead, starting at the hairline medially and laterally to her temples, and ending with small circular friction on the temples **(photo A)**. Repeat this movement, thumbing two or three sen lines **(see illustration)** gradually closer to her eyebrows in the same way. Continue thumbing from the bridge of her nose out along the upper surface of her cheekbone, and then from the nose crease along the lower border of her cheekbone, ending each time with circular friction. Grasp her ear lobes between your thumbs and forefingers and make sensitive circles on the ear pinnae all the way around her ear.

2. PAUSE, IN GRATITUDE

Place your hands lightly along the sides of your partner's face or on her upper chest for three to five breaths, feeling gratitude for the experience you have shared with her. Then bring your hands together in front of your heart and end with another silent or audible "Namaskar." Allow your partner to remain reclining on the mat for as long as she wants to enhance the relaxation and opening effects of the massage, and be sure to offer her a glass of water when she rises from the mat.

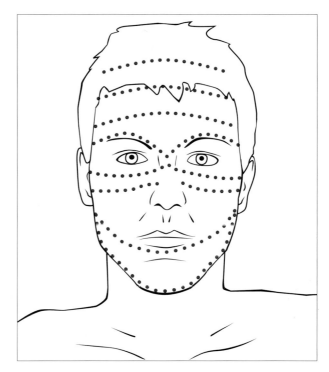

Sen lines on the face

Adaptations for the Physically Challenged

Perform all assisted stretches conservatively to avoid injury or discomfort.

USE PROPS TO ASSIST SEATED STRETCHES

Some people cannot sit comfortably in a cross-legged or extended leg position. To accommodate their needs, you may seat them in a chair and perform the stretches from a standing position (photo A). Depending on your height relative to your partner's height, it may be difficult to lean your body weight into her shoulders to roll the tension out with your forearms. Using props such as two large, sturdy yoga blocks to give yourself enough height will assist you in being able to lean in with your body weight.

To give your partner a good lower back stretch, you may still have her lean forward in the chair with a second chair or a footstool to support her upper body. Some people with low back discomfort will find that a pillow under their knees when they are supine will take some pressure off their back.

LOOK FURTHER TO LEARN MORE

Because Thai massage developed over centuries, there are literally hundreds of sequences, designed to work with the 72,000 sen or energy lines of the body. You do not need to address very many of these lines to perform the basic sequence outlined here, which is serenely powerful in its effects when performed with compassionate intent and focus.

The energetic balancing, conscious connection between giver and receiver, and pleasure of Thai massage all play an important role in supporting wellness. By being passively moved and stretched, a Thai massage receiver surrenders herself to the giver of the massage. Relinquishing control produces a deep relaxation, which in turn bolsters the immune system and may reduce many stress-related conditions.

As you work with a friend or family member repeatedly, you will learn her normal range of motion limitations, and her personal preferences in receiving massage. You will find a wide variation in people's flexibility in different positions, as well as preferences for the massage.

If this form appeals to you, you may want to pursue hands-on education in it. For in-depth training in Thai yoga massage, see www.lotuspalm.com, the website for Kay Thye Chow's Lotus Palm Center and School of Thai Yoga Massage. Courses are offered in Toronto and Montreal, and at various locations in the United States and elsewhere.

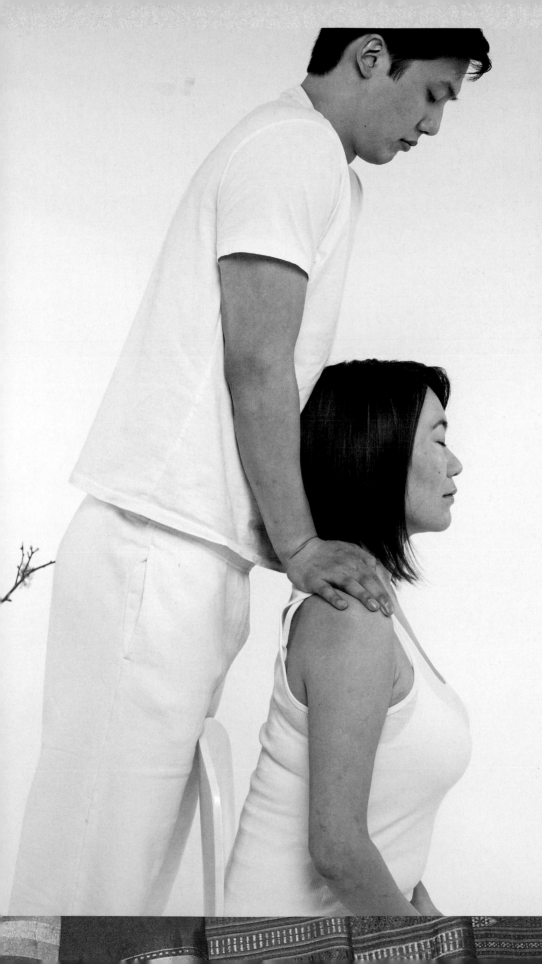

A

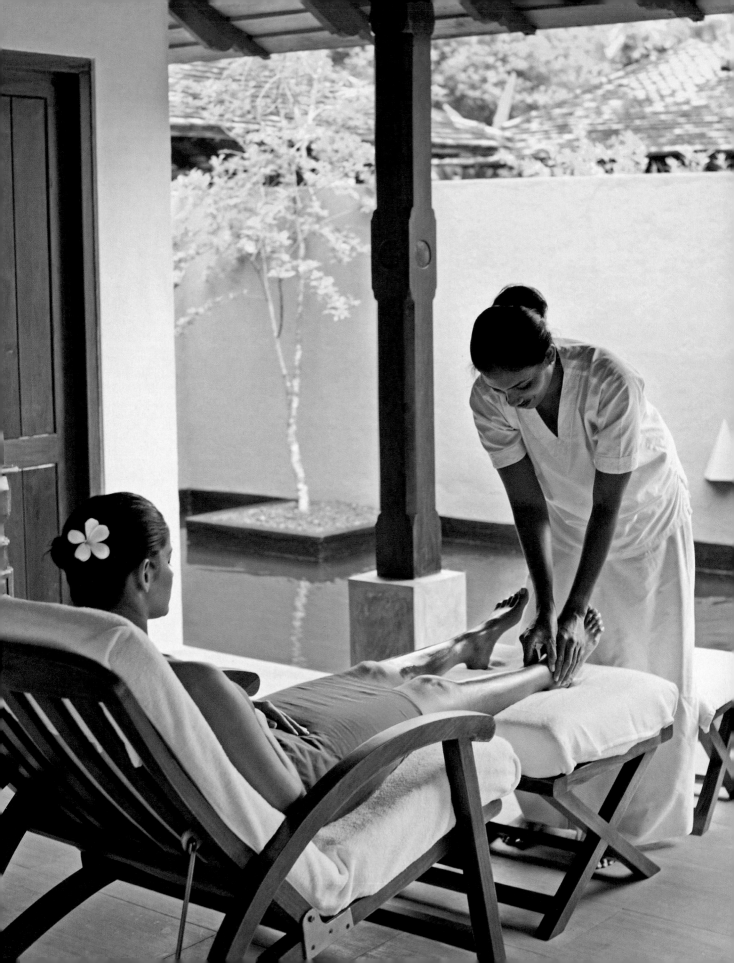

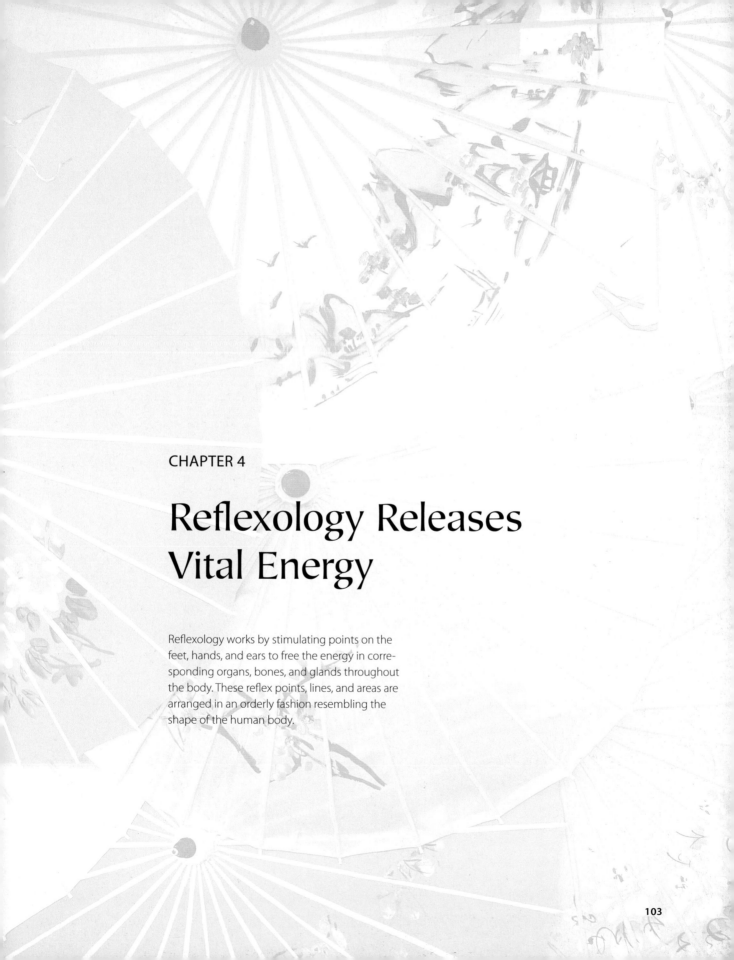

CHAPTER 4

Reflexology Releases Vital Energy

Reflexology works by stimulating points on the feet, hands, and ears to free the energy in corresponding organs, bones, and glands throughout the body. These reflex points, lines, and areas are arranged in an orderly fashion resembling the shape of the human body.

A Map of the Body on the Feet

The body is divided into ten longitudinal reflex zones, with a toe at the end of each line, and five transverse zones, with the front of the feet corresponding to parts above the waist and the back of the feet corresponding to the lower half of the body.

Generally, the ten longitudinal lines go from the head all the way to the toes, with the center lines on the body corresponding to the big toes and the other eight lines moving out to end at the little toes.

The transverse lines cross the feet. The toes correspond to the collarbones, neck, and head; the balls of the feet correspond to the rib cage, and the halfway point on the feet represents the waistline. The heel corresponds to body parts below the waist (see figures 1–3).

The spine reflex area runs down the medial foot, with reflex areas for the arm and shoulder reflected toward the side (see figure 4 on page 112).

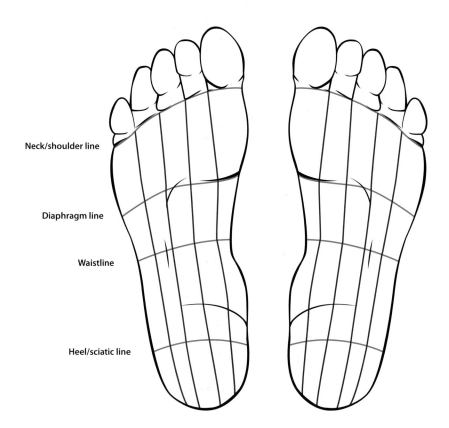

Neck/shoulder line

Diaphragm line

Waistline

Heel/sciatic line

Figure 1. Traverse zones

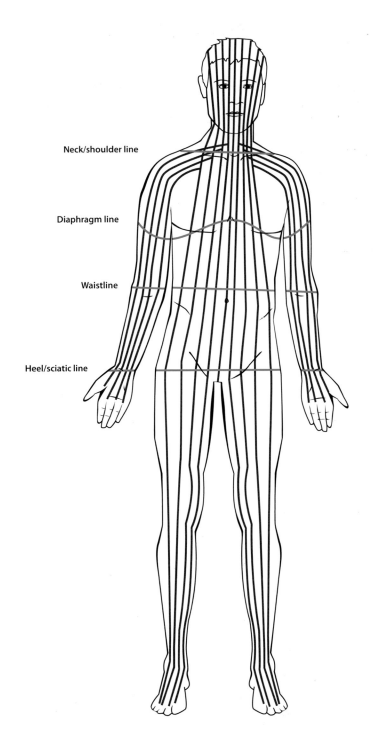

Neck/shoulder line

Diaphragm line

Waistline

Heel/sciatic line

Calm, Clear Intention

Although reflexology is different in its way of working with body systems than most massage, creating a nurturing and calm environment for this practice is just as important as having the clear intention of promoting wellness, balance, and health.

Figure 2. Map of the Body

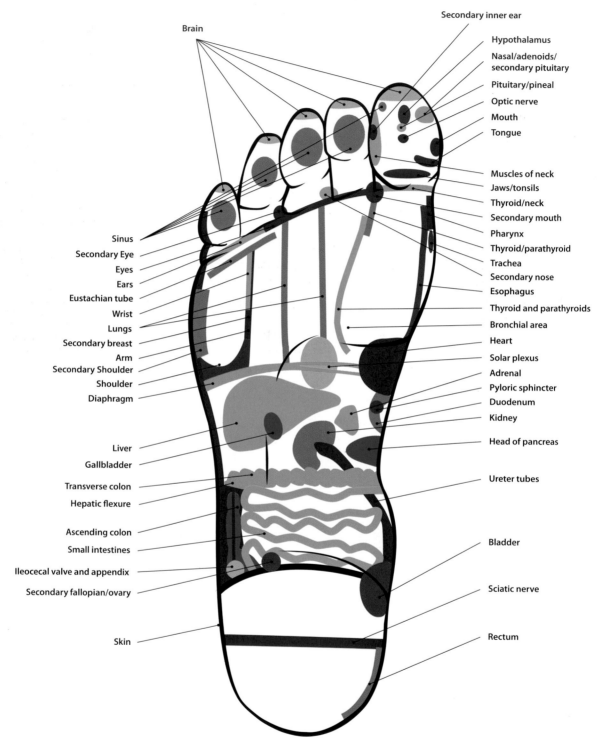

Brain

Secondary inner ear

Hypothalamus

**Nasal/adenoids/
secondary pituitary**

Pituitary/pineal

Optic nerve

Mouth

Tongue

Muscles of neck

Jaws/tonsils

Thyroid/neck

Secondary mouth

Pharynx

Thyroid/parathyroid

Trachea

Secondary nose

Esophagus

Thyroid and parathyroids

Bronchial area

Heart

Solar plexus

Adrenal

Pyloric sphincter

Duodenum

Kidney

Head of pancreas

Ureter tubes

Bladder

Sciatic nerve

Rectum

Sinus

Secondary Eye

Eyes

Ears

Eustachian tube

Wrist

Lungs

Secondary breast

Arm

Secondary Shoulder

Shoulder

Diaphragm

Liver

Gallbladder

Transverse colon

Hepatic flexure

Ascending colon

Small intestines

Ileocecal valve and appendix

Secondary fallopian/ovary

Skin

Figure 3. Plantar reflexes of the right foot

Pressure and Length of Holds in Reflexology

Press each point firmly for a few seconds to stimulate the nervous system to release tension. The feet essentially have no fatty tissue, so take care to press conservatively on this area, where so many small bones, tendons, connective tissue, and ligaments are close to the surface. If it appears that your partner's feet and ankles are fat, press firmly into the swollen tissue and see if an indentation remains for more than ten seconds. If it does, you should discontinue the work because the indentation may indicate pitting edema, a type of swelling associated with severe circulatory problems. Use slightly more than the amount of pressure it takes to press the average elevator button and you'll be exerting an appropriate amount of pressure to use in reflexology.

Reflexologists believe that a "vital energy" circulates among the organs in the human body and penetrates into every living cell. Whenever this energy is blocked, the reflex zone can indicate where blockages exist in different organs. Therefore, if someone has a problem in a particular organ, pressing on the corresponding reflex point or area may cause the person to experience some pain, but the organ or body area will move toward better function and balance.

**Warning!
See a Doctor
for Foot Injury**

Reflexology is recommended as a complementary therapy which encourages overall healing and should not replace medical treatment. If you have foot ulcers, a foot injury, or blood vessel disease such as blood clots or if you are pregnant, consult your doctor before having reflexology. The sequences detailed in this chapter are indicated for wellness; seek the services of a certified reflexologist if you have specific conditions you wish to treat with reflexology.

Relaxation Sequence

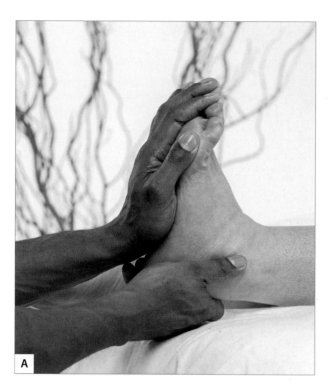

A

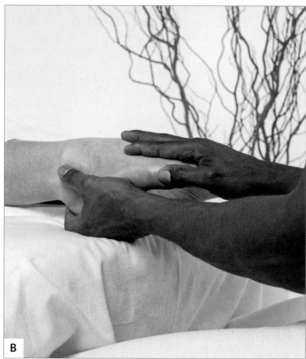

B

Many different reflexology sequences are aimed at balancing different systems and organs, and the following relaxation sequence is a good precursor to the next stress-relieving sequence. Most of us in today's fast-paced world can use the half-hour to forty-minute mini vacation with our feet up! You will need a rolling chair, a stool, or a balance ball that is high enough to allow you to work on your partner's feet without having to either elevate your shoulders or bend forward. The ideal position in which to work is with your feet flat on the floor and your torso erect.

1. FLEX THE FOOT AND ROTATE THE ANKLE

Begin by holding one of your partner's feet in each hand, and as she starts to relax, feel your skin temperatures come together. Then hold her right foot at the heel with your right hand and use your left hand to first press the ball of her foot up toward her head by leaning into it with your left hand; this movement is called dorsiflexion (**photo A**). Lean back, bringing her forefoot down toward you in plantar flexion (**photo B**), and repeat the back-and-forth movement several times, not forcing movement but encouraging full range in the ankle.

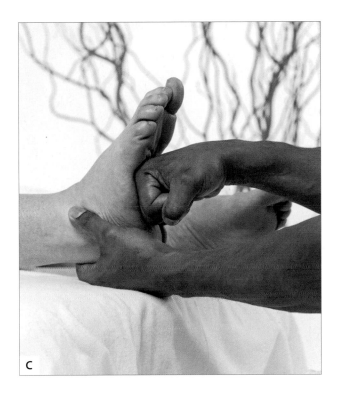

C

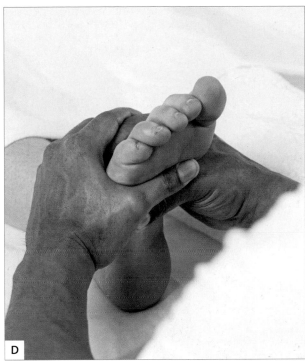

D

While holding her foot in this position, add circular movement so that you are rotating her ankle both clockwise and counterclockwise. You may notice cracking, popping, or grinding noises as you take the ankle through its range of motion, but unless it is uncomfortable for your partner, the noises are not a problem. Rotate the ankle three times in each direction or until you feel it is moving smoothly through its range of motion. Then, with your hand in a loose fist, draw the knuckles from the heel to the toes a few times, covering the entire sole of the foot (**photo C**).

2. WAG THE SOLE, SQUEEZE THE FOOT

Place your hands on each side of your partner's foot, near the ball, and slowly turn the sole of her foot inward (inversion) with enough pressure to move the side to its natural limit in range of motion from your right hand; then move the foot outward (eversion) with your left hand. As you get a feel for the range of motion of her ankle in these directions, you may move the foot more quickly back and forth.

With your fingers on the dorsal surface and your thumbs on the sole, hold the foot firmly and squeeze it with your whole hand on each of your exhalations, moving your thumbs inward to pass each other at the midline of the sole of the foot (**photo D**). Begin at the front of the foot and gradually move toward the heel. Do not slide your hands down the foot but rather keep repositioning them to make passes inward.

Great Chairs for Reflexology

Your partner should be comfortably reclining, with a small pillow under her head and neck or a rolled towel supporting her neck. The zero-gravity chair is particularly good for reflexology. A similar lawn chair or even a standard living room recliner would also work since the receiver's legs should be elevated above the hips for a session.

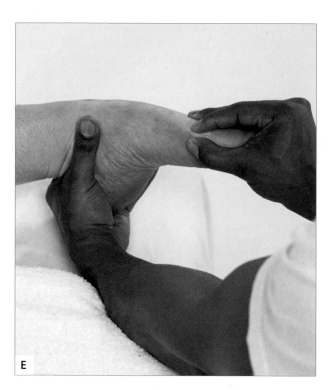

E

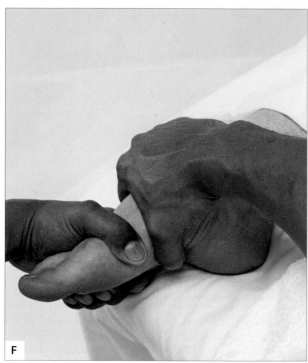

F

3. PINCH AND WRING THE SPINAL REFLEX LINE

Holding your partner's heel in your left hand, make pinching type movements (but gentler), moving your thumb and forefinger toward each other along the spinal reflex line on the medial arch of her foot **(photo E)**. Start at the big toe with your thumb on its plantar surface and your index finger on the dorsal surface, and work all the way to the front of the heel, then back up to the big toe. Wrap your hands around her foot, with your thumbs on the spinal reflex line (medial arch), and wring the foot by squeezing it and rotating your hands in opposite directions, moving up and down the foot **(photo F)**. Your partner may feel a loosening or warmth in her vertebral column as a result of these actions.

Spinal Reflex Line

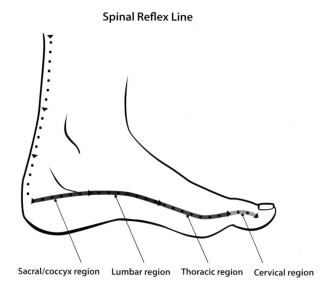

Sacral/coccyx region   Lumbar region   Thoracic region   Cervical region

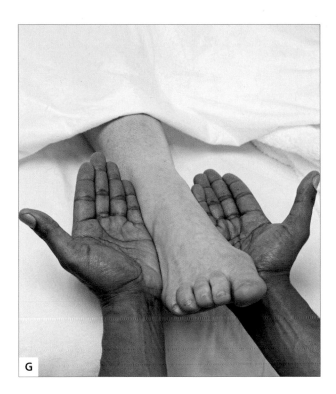

G

4. ROCK THE FOOT, LIFT THE TOES

Holding your partner's heel between your hands, with your palms facing up, vigorously move your palms forward and back (photo G). This will cause the forefoot to rock back and forth loosely and will warm the heel. With your left hand, hold all of your partner's toes and lift them up, lengthening them away from the heel.

Natural Healing

The medical profession traditionally scoffed at claims made for reflexology's effectiveness, but the National Center for Complementary and Alternative Medicine (NCCAM) has deemed it a true integrative health treatment, having immediate and long-term effects on disease, quality of life, and bodily function. Ongoing studies, many of which have been conducted in China and Europe, have verified the following benefits:

- Relaxation and stress relief
- Reduction in migraine and tension headaches
- Improvement in kidney function
- Improvement in geriatric activities of daily living
- Improvement in blood flow and reduction of high blood pressure
- Improved serum cholesterol levels
- Pain reduction, including post-surgical pain
- Reduction in symptoms of PMS
- Faster post-operative recovery
- Reduction of nausea, anxiety, and pain associated with cancer treatments and improvement in perceived quality of life during those treatments
- Increased blood flow to digestive organs and relief of constipation
- Improvement in type II diabetes symptoms
- Decreased pain in some forms of arthritis
- Improvement in sleep quality and more rapid recovery from fatigue and muscle soreness in athletes; reduction of insomnia
- Useful in some cases for phantom limb sensation reduction
- Helpful for anxiety, depression, and post-traumatic stress disorder
- Supportive in labor, delivery, and lactation
- Ease of discomforts of tired feet

Warning!
Crystals Blasting

The fleeting discomfort upon touch of a reflex point theoretically originates from crystal congestion or imbalance in the reflex zone. Reflexology can break down the crystals and result in pain or dysfunction relief by removing the energy blocks and thus decongesting the affected zones.

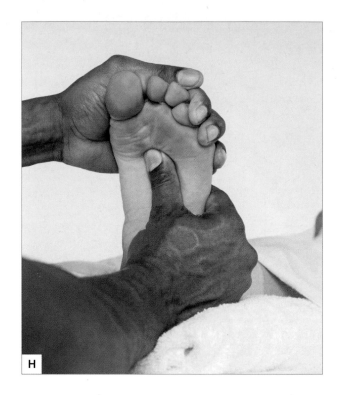

5. PRESS YOUR THUMB AND PULL THE FOOT OVER

Place your right thumb on the diaphragm line below your partner's big toe and pull his forefoot toward your thumb, gently intensifying the pressure of your thumb by moving his foot over it (photo H). With each of your exhalations, press your thumb along points on the diaphragm line toward the lateral side of your partner's foot, bringing the foot toward your thumb on each point. Bring your thumb back to the center of the diaphragm line, press in, and bring the foot over once more, asking your partner to inhale and hold the breath for a moment. Release this point, the solar plexus point, as your partner slowly exhales.

6. PULL THE LOWER LEG TO RELAX THE BACK, HIP, AND KNEE

If your partner's knee is flexed, place a pillow under his lower leg to fully extend the leg in a relaxed position. Hold his heel in one hand and with the other, hold his upper calf, just below the knee. Lean back and exert a long, slow pull on the heel while you have him breathe deeply (photo I). This completes the relaxation sequence by relaxing the back, hip, and knee areas.

7. REPEAT THE RELAXATION SEQUENCE ON THE LEFT FOOT

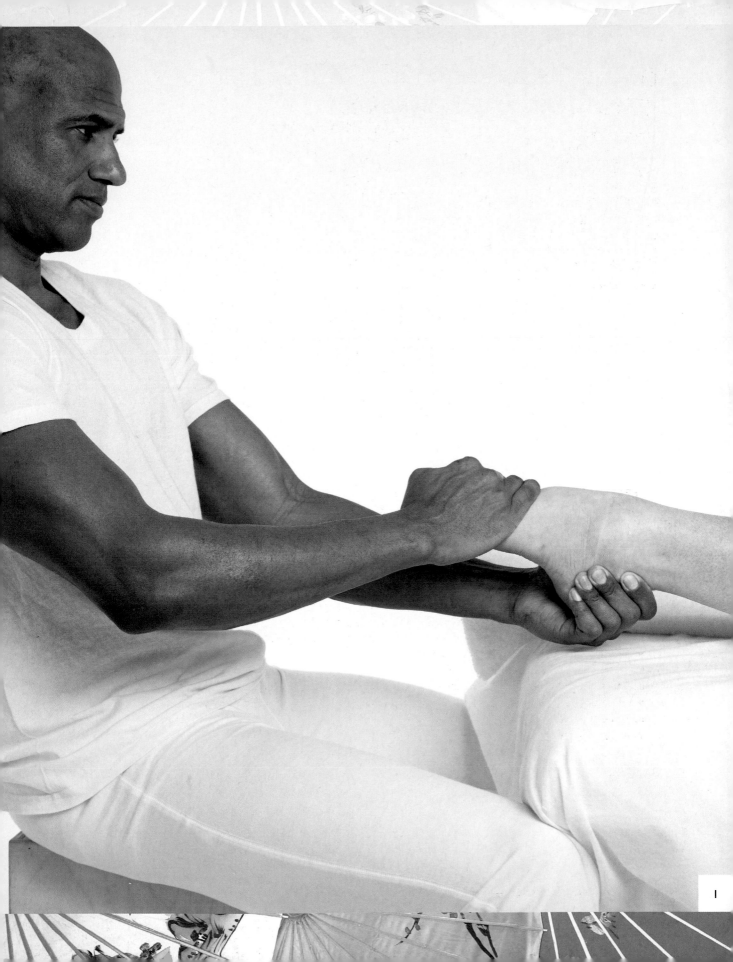

Stress-Relieving Sequence

Even though we tend to feel stress as a condition of the nervous system, there are a host of physiological components to it. Addressing the effects of stress on the body is helpful in preventing long-term damage on the body's systems. As you stimulate points in the following sequence, try to coordinate the pressing of your fingers with your breath.

TAKE YOUR HANDS FOR A WALK

A couple of techniques are important to try before you begin this sequence:

Thumb walking can be practiced by placing your thumb on either your opposite forearm or your thigh. Flex your thumb so that the last joint is perpendicular to the tissue. Press directly down through the tip; then allow the joint to extend, still keeping some downward pressure. As you again flex your thumb joint to come up on the tip, you will notice your thumb has traveled a tiny distance forward. As you repeat this move several times, you will notice how the thumb rocks slightly as it moves forward (**photo A**).

Finger walking is the same movement practiced with one or more fingers at the same time. Circling is used by placing the tip of the thumb directly on a reflex point and making tiny rotations not moving over the skin, but rather more like a gentle drilling inward (**photo B**). Unless noted otherwise, circle clockwise on women and counterclockwise on men.

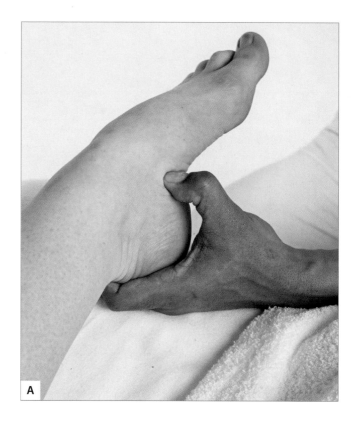

A

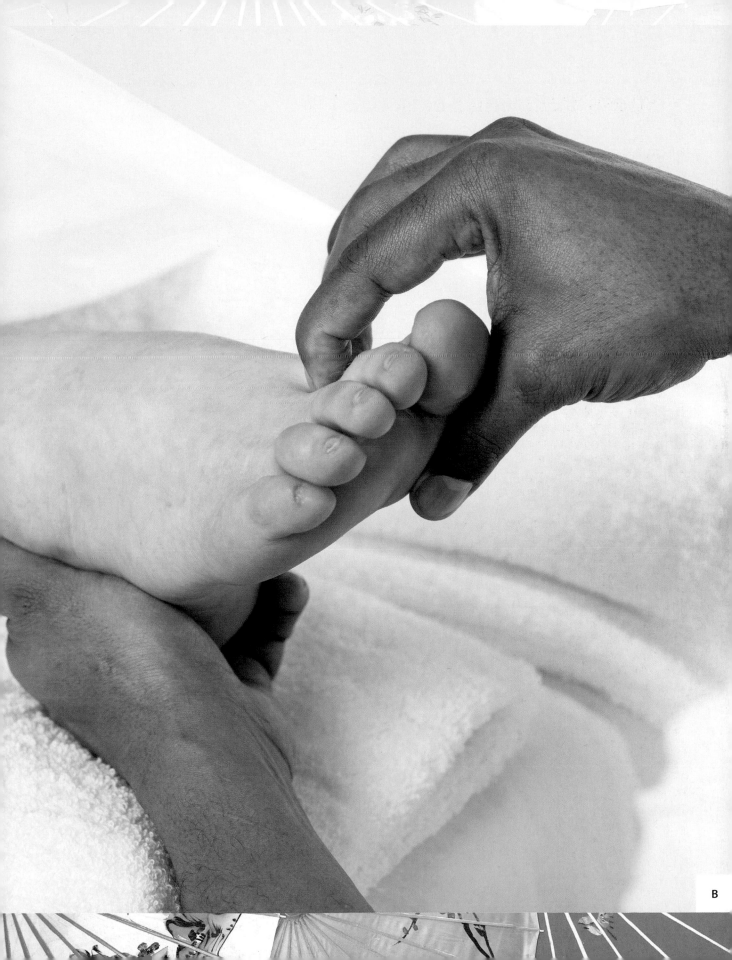

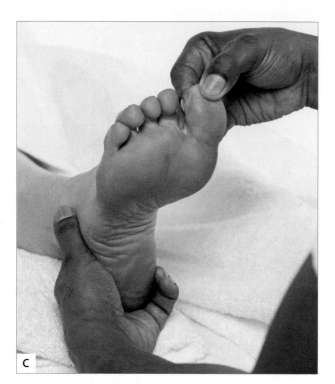

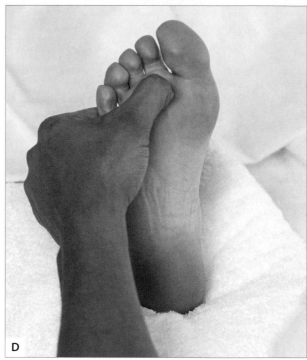

1. PRESS FOR SEVEN COUNTS, SEVEN TIMES

In this sequence, perform each action on your partner's left foot, then his right foot, seven times each. Begin by repeating the diaphragm line presses and press the solar plexus point from the relaxation sequence. Hold for a count of seven or nine. This will enhance the open breathing you have established with the relaxation sequence and will signal the abdominal organs and muscles to relax.

2. PRESS THE PITUITARY POINT IN THE BIG TOE

Press into your partner's pituitary gland reflex point, which is in the center of the widest part of the plantar surface of the big toe (photo C). You may circle here as well for several counts. Stimulate the point firmly seven times on each foot, producing a calming sensation.

3. STIMULATE THE PARATHYROID REFLEX

Moving from the medial base of your partner's big toe to the other side of the toe, walk your thumb across the crease on the plantar surface where the toe joins the foot (the thyroid reflex [photo D]) and follow with thumb presses from the base of the ball of the foot between the first and second metatarsal bones up to the end point of the thyroid reflex seven times; this is the parathyroid reflex (photo E). Stimulating these gland reflex areas may enhance tranquility in the body.

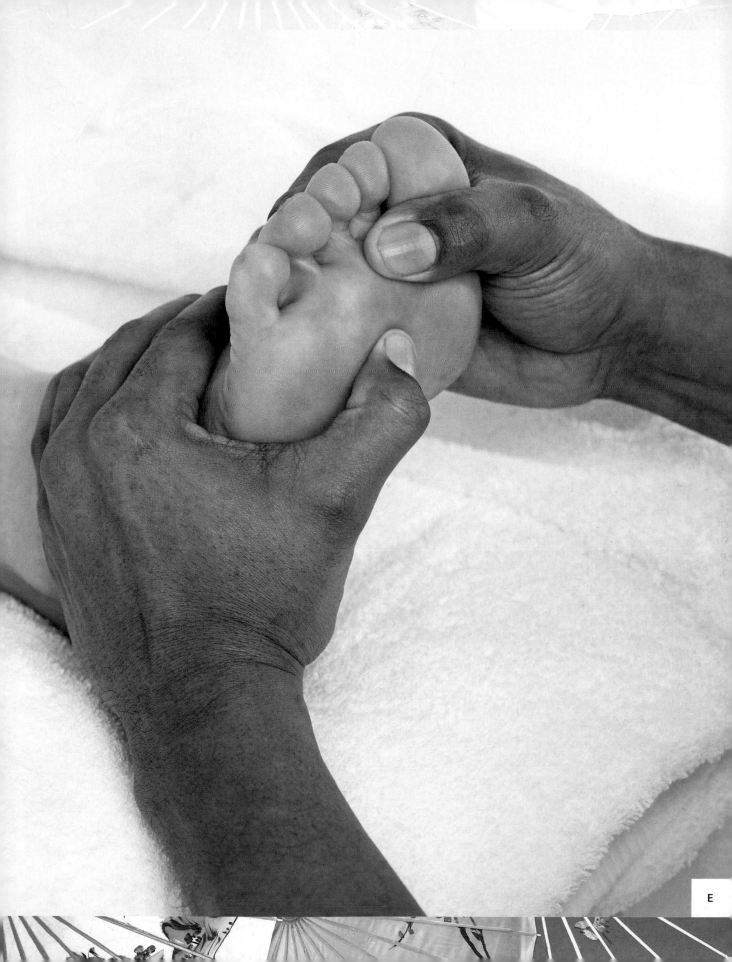

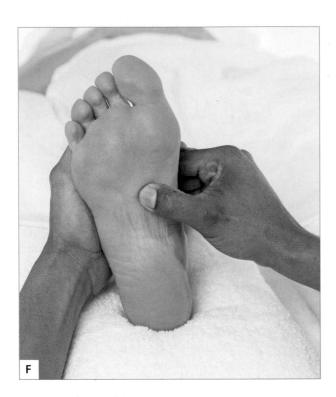

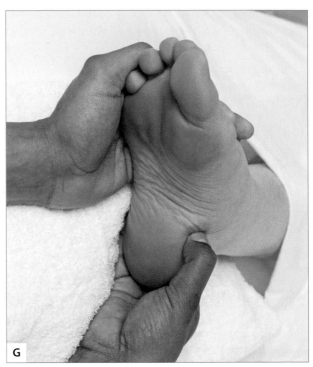

4. NURTURE THE LUNGS AND ENLIVEN THE TISSUES

The lung reflex consists of two lines running from the diaphragm line on the sole of the foot up to the base of the medial and lateral sides of the middle toes. Thumb-walk up each line from the diaphragm line to your partner's toes (**photo F**); you may also follow the same pattern on the top, or dorsal, surface of the foot as a helper reflex. Nurturing the lungs helps to increase the oxygen level in the blood, enlivening the tissues throughout the body.

5. BALANCE THE BODY'S FLUIDS WITH THE KIDNEY REFLEX

The kidney reflex relates to stabilizing or lowering blood pressure. There are two ways to stimulate it. You may either thumb-walk the area on the plantar surface of your partner's feet that is bisected by the waistline line across the foot, or you can place your entire thumb on the bean-shaped kidney reflex with your thumb crossing the waistline and circle, press, and hold (**photo G**). In addition, you may start at the bladder reflex, which is at the medial edge of the sole of the foot just forward of the abdominal cavity line near the heel, and thumb-walk up through the urinary reflexes, including the bladder and ureter reflexes, on your way to stimulating the kidney reflex, which is more toward the center of the feet.

6. THUMB-WALK ALONG THE SPINAL REFLEX

The spine reflex soothes (see page 112) and calms nervous responses in the spinal cord. This is a very important center, as thirty-one sets of peripheral spinal nerves exit from the spinal cord and connect all the organs, glands, and regions of the body, providing sensory, motor (movement), and integrative (the interface of

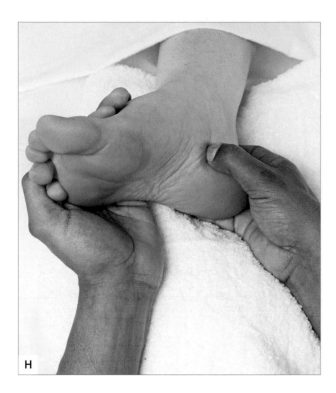

H

Ancient and Recent History of Reflexology

Because reflexology is an ancient practice, its origin and history are difficult to track. It is thought to have been passed down through oral tradition and was possibly first recorded as a pictograph on an Egyptian tomb in 2330 BCE. Cultures in China, Japan, India, Europe, and North and South America were also known to have used the hands and feet to affect the rest of the body.

In 1917, a physician named William Fitzgerald developed zone therapy. He found that by applying pressure to a zone that corresponded to an injury location, he could relieve pain during minor surgical procedures. He divided the body into ten vertical zones ending in the fingers and toes, noting that pressure on one part of the zone could affect everything else within that zone. Dr. Shelby Riley expanded on Fitzgerald's work by developing maps of horizontal body zones that correspond with reflex points on the feet and hands. Eunice Ingham, a physiotherapist, refined both of their works in the 1930s, finding the feet to have the most effective reflex points, and developed the standard foot maps that are in use today.

Theory holds that the 72,000 sensory nerves in the feet are key in the body's immediate reflexive "fight or flight" response to danger, communicating with all the internal organs to cause sudden responses like an adrenaline surge.

sensory and motor) functions for the body. The spine reflex runs along the medial longitudinal arches of the feet from the medial edge of the big toes all the way back to the medial heels, its line arching parallel to the arch of the sole of the foot. Begin to thumb-walk directly below your partner's ankle bone (the medial malleolis) **(photo H)** and stimulate the spine reflex all the way to the medial edge of his big toenail. As you thumb-walk forward on his foot, you will be stimulating points in the spinal cord increasingly close to his head.

7. REPEAT THE DIAPHRAGM AND SOLAR PLEXUS PRESSES

Repeat the diaphragm line presses, as well as the solar plexus point with which you began the sequence, to again enhance open and relaxed breathing.

Chakra Sequence

In the Indian tradition, chakras are spinning energy vortexes related to consciousness—part of the subtle anatomy of the body, a field of energy. Each chakra is associated with a specific endocrine gland or glands. Energetic balancing goes hand in hand with hormonal balancing, leading to enhanced vitality and youthful vigor.

Root chakra—Gonads/ovaries
Sacral chakra—Adrenal gland
Solar plexus—Pancreas
Heart chakra—Thymus
Throat chakra—Thyroid and parathyroid
glands
Third-eye chakra—Pituitary gland

FINDING CHAKRAS ON THE FEET

The chakra system is located along the spinal reflex at the medial side of both feet from the big toe to the ankle and in the hands from the thumb to the wrist. There are two ways to balance chakras on the feet. The first is to stimulate points on the toes, and the second is to stimulate the chakra points along the spinal reflex.

1. INFUSE THE TOES WITH COLOR

Begin with your partner seated or lying supine. Hold the same toes of each foot firmly for as long as you desire or until you feel your partner has had enough, usually between thirty seconds and one minute. Send the appropriate color to each toe or finger (see the "Color Your World" sidebar). A deep sigh or yawn is a signal that a release or a change has occurred, and you can continue to the next toe or finger. Become aware of the sense of peace and harmony that affects both of you.

2. HOLD, STROKE, PULSE, OR VIBRATE THE CHAKRAS

Hold the same chakra on each foot simultaneously using either your thumb or two fingers. Send the chakra color or ask your partner to breathe in that color. Hold, stroke, pulse, or vibrate the chakra point until you feel a shift. The shift may occur when you or your partner sigh or yawn or when you feel an energy or vibration in your hands or body. Hold each spot with either your thumb or index and middle fingers.

3. CREATE A HARMONIOUS LINK

Finish by linking the root chakra at the heel and the crown chakra at the top of the big toe for physical and spiritual harmony, holding each point simultaneously. This completes a chakra session on the feet. For some people, it can cause striking changes in how they feel; for others it may be so subtle that they are consciously unaware of any effects. Regardless of the global adjustments in the body/mind, you should notice a level of peace and relaxation, not only in your partner but also in yourself, after performing this sequence.

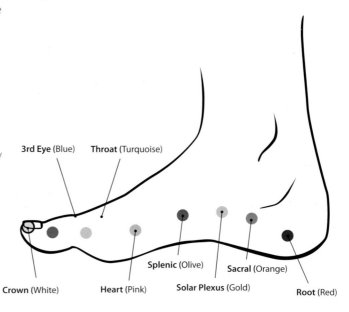

3rd Eye (Blue)   Throat (Turquoise)

Splenic (Olive)

Sacral (Orange)

Crown (White)   Heart (Pink)   Solar Plexus (Gold)   Root (Red)

Color Your World

Each toe and finger has its own chakra and color:

a. The pinky toe and finger relate to the root chakra and are red.

b. The fourth toe and ring finger relate to the sacral chakra and are orange.

c. The middle toe and finger reflect the solar plexus chakra and are yellow.

d. The second toe and index finger involve the heart chakra and are green or pink.

e. The neck of the big toe and thumb relate to the throat chakra and are blue.

f. The top joint of the big toe and thumb refer to the brow and the crown chakra and are indigo and violet.

The root chakra—On the heel of both feet, below the ankle, medial side, in a slight depression in the foot

The sacral chakra—On the medial side at the navicular bone, where the heel joins the arch of the foot

The solar plexus chakra—On the end of the metatarsal bone

The heart chakra—At the head of the metatarsal bone

The throat chakra—In the proximal joint of the big toe; the "neck" of the big toe

The third eye chakra—On the bump on the medial side of the big toe

The crown chakra—At the top of the big toe

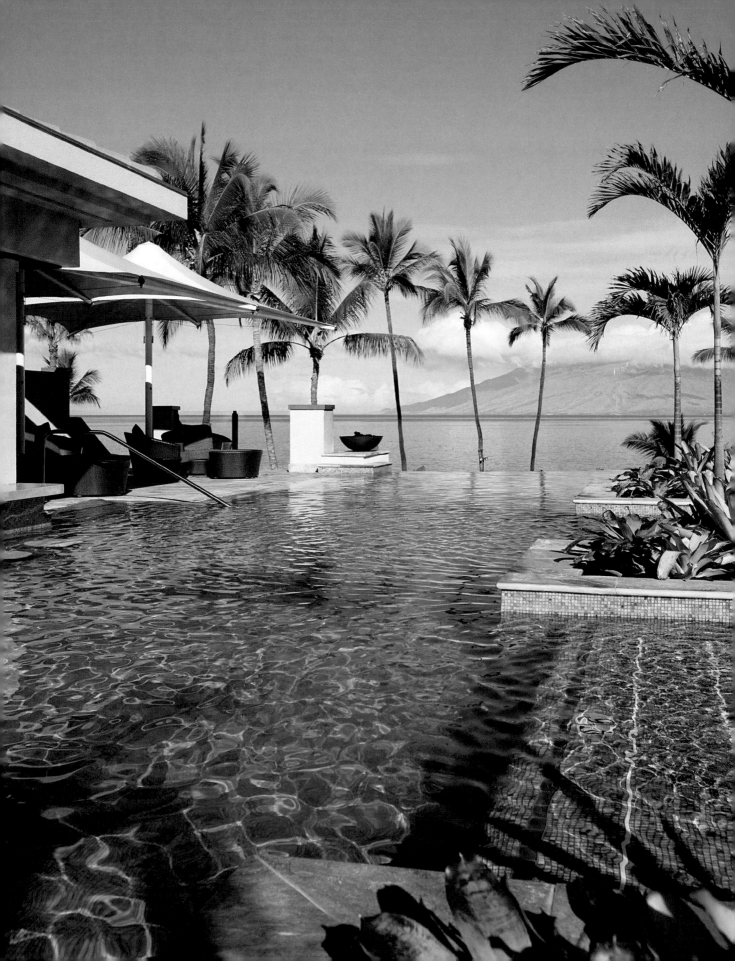

CHAPTER 5

Lomi Lomi Spirals Love and Harmony

The word lomi lomi means massage, or "to weave love." Lomi lomi is based on the Hawaiian philosophy of Huna—that everything in the universe seeks harmony, love, and balance. Lomi lomi is considered to be a moving prayer, used to restore fluidity and balance in a person's being with the use of continuous, flowing strokes which nurture the body and soul.

Traditionally, lomi lomi was performed on a handwoven grass mat on the floor, but today massage tables are usually used for sessions which range from forty-five minutes to a few hours, as in the case of ritual life transition preparations by Hawaiian healers, or kahunas.

Lomi lomi is performed with minimal draping of the receiver to facilitate bodywork on large portions of the body and generally is performed with a heavy application of oil, sometimes including essential oils. Ideally, lomi lomi engages the receiver in the process by having him breathe deeply and inviting positive thoughts and emotions into his being during the session.

Preparation for Lomi Lomi

The receiver should avoid eating a heavy meal or drinking alcohol in the hours leading up to the lomi lomi session. Given the number of hula movements involved in giving lomi lomi massage, the giver might want to follow the same guidelines!

Set up your massage table in a serene location, preferably with candles and flowers in the room to remind you of the sacred essence of Huna. Generally, oil is used liberally in lomi lomi, so have a plastic squeeze bottle or a bowl of oil warmed to at least room temperature and make sure the receiver knows that he may be well greased, including his hair, following the session. This is not the sort of bodywork one would want to receive and then return to the office, unless a shower is available. You may choose to use small amounts of essential oils in your base oil: Ylang-ylang relaxes the muscles and has a sedative and aphrodisiac effect; rosemary and marjoram oils are beneficial for muscle aches and headaches.

Use a twin-size fitted sheet on the massage table that you don't mind getting oily or have some oil-removing laundry treatment on hand and wash the sheet and draping towel immediately following use. Letting the oil set in will increase the likelihood of staining and cause a rancid smell in the cloth. Have a bath towel or a hand towel for use as a drape or dispense with draping altogether. Just be sure the room where you will have the session is nice and warm.

Lomi lomi usually begins with your partner lying face down, or prone, on the table. Commence with a few moments of stillness with your hands palm up to receive universal energy or resting lightly on his back, transmitting energy and establishing connection. During this brief stillness, a traditional lomi lomi practitioner would say or chant a blessing or prayer, asking for whatever healing is needed. You might choose to work in the traditional way, voicing a prayer or chant audibly or silently, as long as your intent is to promote balance, harmony, and well-being.

Lava, the Original Hot Stone

Once you have gotten a feel for the movements and sequence of a lomi lomi massage, you can integrate hot stones into a session, using them as tools. Hawaiians had access to lava rock and traditionally used it in healing massage sessions.

Set Your Intention

Intention is the key to the practice of lomi lomi, as it is in most forms of bodywork; whatever internal or spiritual setting of intention helps you to maintain your focus on the healing benefits you seek for your partner is perfect for your use.

The Moves, Strokes, and Pressure of Lomi Lomi

- Hula movements, with rhythmic spiraling movements of the hips, forearms, and hands, fluidly penetrate and create gentle waves all over the body. Different parts of the body may be massaged at the same time, which assists the receiver in relaxing totally.
- Figure eights and spirals result from your hands following the movement of your hips in a hula fashion.
- Gentle stretches of the body and easy joint rotations assist the release of tension and enhance the flow of energy.
- Lomi lomi is all about flowing movement rather than seeking to exert depth and pressure. All the moves should be fluid and superficial, skimming the surface of the body only firmly enough that ticklishness is not elicited from the touch.

Lomi Lomi Prone Sequence

Before you start moving your hands on your partner's back, remember that the session may be slow and relaxing or faster and more invigorating, depending on how your partner's body responds and whether his goal for the session is to be relaxed or invigorated. It may be useful occasionally as you massage to remind your partner to give himself permission to let go. Invite him to breathe in and accept relaxation, joy, and inner peace.

1. WALK YOUR PALMS ON THE BACK
   Standing at the head of the table, before adding oil to your hands, walk your palms down your partner's back, shifting weight onto your left foot and left hand simultaneously, then to the right (**photo A**). See if you can get some hula figure eights started in your hips as you perform this cat walking down each side of his spine, never working directly on the vertebrae, and leaning with even pressure from the heel of each hand through the fingertips. Integrate some outward circular flaring motions with each compression. Return from his lower back to his shoulders in the same way.

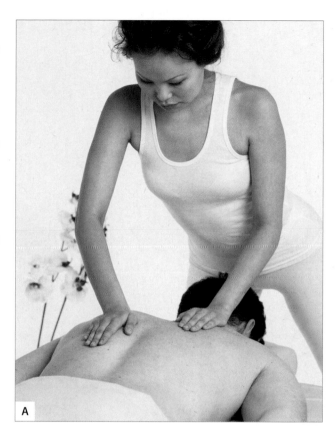

A

Put on Hawaiian Music and Remember to Hula!

Playing Hawaiian or other flowing music during a lomi lomi session is a nice touch and makes it easier to keep hula-type movements going as you perform the massage. It may be helpful before the session to take some time to move with the music, making figure eights with your hips as you bring your arms up while inhaling and floating your arms back down while exhaling and then moving your hips from side to side and in circles, gradually moving your whole body to the music. You should feel intensified energy throughout your body after you have moved with the music for a few minutes, which indicates you are ready to transmit this energy to your partner. Lomi lomi is a flowing form of bodywork, and the movements need to come from your entire energized self.

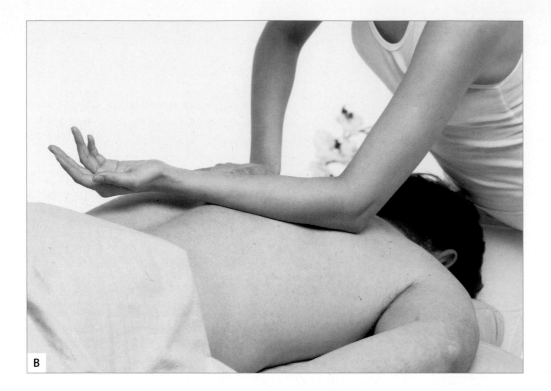

B

Add Oil and Move in Figure Eights

Still standing at the head of the table, add an abundance of oil to your hands and blow into them; in lomi lomi this is considered to be breathing life into the hands. Spread the oil on your partner's back and begin making alternating figure eights with your forearms, rotating your palms skyward as you glide your forearms toward your partner's hips **(photo B)** and rotating your palms down toward his body as you glide your forearms back toward yourself **(photo C)**. Get into the rhythmic motion with your entire body, allowing your body weight to "fall in" to the tissue with control. Using the figure eights superficially, you may cross the spine, but never put the pressure of your weight on the vertebrae. Almost all of the pressure you exert in lomi lomi is pushing away; very little is pulling back toward your own body, even when the strokes are flowing back toward you.

Channel Energy and Do the Healing Dance

Imagine that you are spiraling energy into your partner's body, breaking up tension, layer by layer. Allow your partner to integrate what you are offering him by pausing from time to time. Some practitioners use a raised hand to channel energy down to focus and stay in touch with the light, all the while placing a stationary hand on the receiver. Using your entire body as you apply strokes will help remind you that lomi lomi is a healing dance. When the tissue feels looser and lighter after layers are released, you can move into deeper movements. Lomi lomi pressure can range from very superficial to deep and from slow to fast. Check in with your partner about the amount of pressure you are using and the speed with which you are massaging.

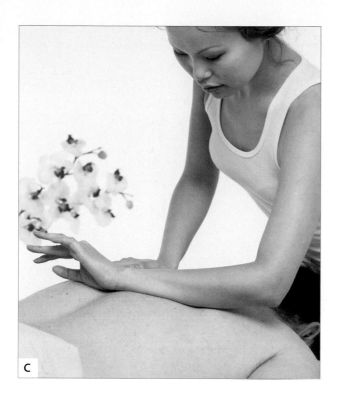

C

The Center of Strength

For all strokes in lomi lomi, but especially for the long strokes, movement should come from your center. Inhale energy from the universe and exhale it through your arms as you spiral or glide each stroke into your partner's body. Let your body initiate the movement, rather than just using your arm strength; it makes a huge difference in how cohesive and integrated the strokes will feel to the receiver. Shift your weight from your back foot to your front foot and maintain attention on the point of contact into your partner's body so that you can get behind your strokes and maintain focus.

Benefits of Lomi Lomi

- Releases trapped tension and relieves stress
- Promotes enhanced blood and lymph flow
- Stimulates the elimination of waste and toxins
- Promotes a sense of rejuvenation of the body, mind, spirit, and emotions
- May enhance a sense of peace, harmony, and well-being
- Leads to a more dynamic life-energy flow, which may be blocked by ideas or beliefs as much as by muscle tension
- Enhances immune response
- Decompresses joints
- May restore an expanded sense of self

2. MOVE FROM YOUR CENTER TO AWAKEN THE SPINE

Move into using your whole hand, from heels and palms to supported fingers, to awaken the spine, with the vertebrae between the index and middle fingers of one hand and your other hand supporting your fingers moving directly down your partner's back to his hips **(photo D)**. Follow with more loosening forearm spiraling strokes. Remember to perform somewhere between three and six strokes to allow your partner to relax but not to be irritated by receiving the same stroke too many times.

Build Heat with a Sawing Stroke

To create more heat and energy in the back muscles, use Madam Pele's Special: longitudinal friction applied using the ulnar, or pinky side, of your hands and forearms in a sawing motion parallel to the spine. The faster you apply this forearm friction stroke, the more heat you will create, and the motion of your forearms moving in opposite directions will confuse the back muscles into letting go while the heat enhances the warming effect of the friction. You can continue with this forearm friction until you feel the back muscles soften or until your arms tire from the sawing motion. Keep your hands relaxed or your forearms will feel rigid rather than yielding.

3. MAKE CIRCLES AND SPIRALS ON THE BACK AND HIPS

Move to the left side of the table and perform figure-eight strokes from the side of your partner's lower back upward toward his shoulders, gliding with the fleshy part of the ulna, and take out the slack in the tissue **(photo E)**. These rolling strokes may be short or long up the left side of your partner's back. Bring your right forearm back to your partner's hip and perform figure eights around the bone, followed by light spirals with your elbow around the hip. Although you want to be leaning into the movements, you do not want to lean heavily or exert a great deal of pressure. Lomi lomi as described here is fairly superficial

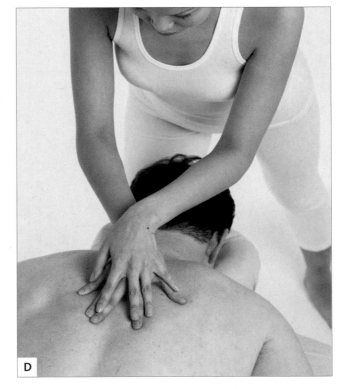

D

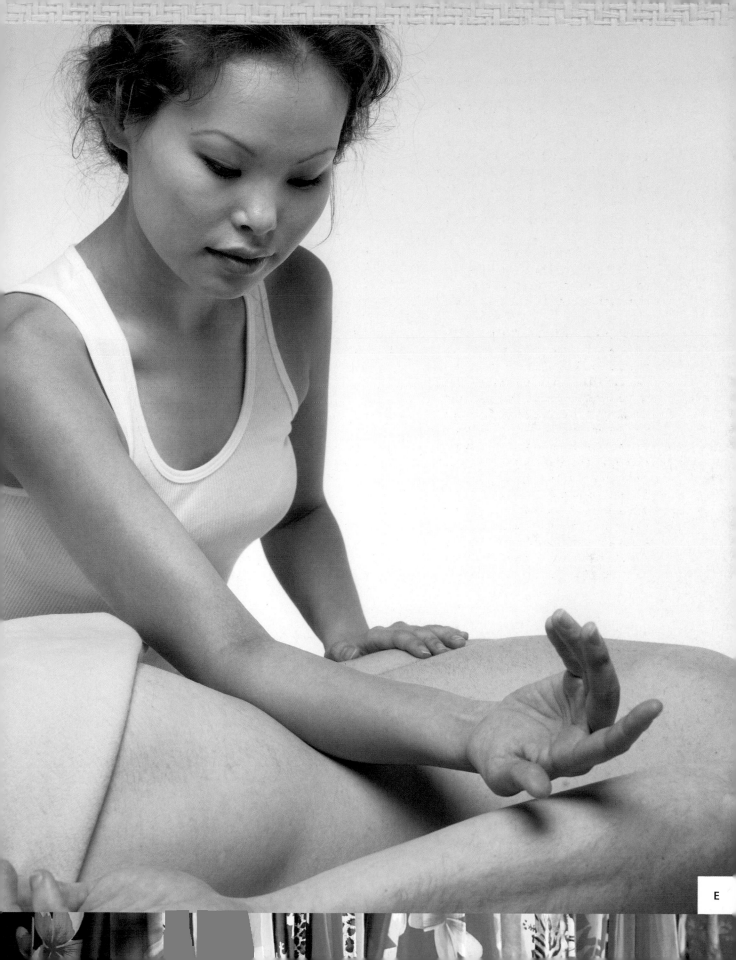

bodywork, and your partner should not feel effort from you but should feel a light dancing quality of your arms. Circles and spirals around the hip can help to release held tension from too much sitting or driving and reduce the discomfort that can come from tight muscles.

Glide Your Forearm along the Body

Repeat rolling motions up your partner's back with your forearm, facing his head. As you lightly spiral around his scapula, move to face his feet and continue the rolling action down his left arm to his hand and back to his shoulder. Your hips should always be pointed in the direction of the strokes you are making. Switch arms and scoop his upper shoulder muscles, the trapezius, with your left forearm; while leaning in, glide your forearm all the way down the left side of his back, close to but not on his spine. Continue the gliding stroke with your forearm all the way down his leg. Lighten the pressure behind his ankle, in the area of the Achilles tendon, and glide your forearm down the sole of his foot before rotating to face his head; then glide back up his leg and thigh, pausing at the hip.

Soft Fists, Warm Heart

Your hands should feel soft; a tight fist will feel aggressive and uncomfortable to your partner and may leave your hands achy after the massage.

Aloha: Love and Energy

Aloha spirit is an integral part of the massage. Aloha's deeper meaning is "the joyful sharing of life energy in the present" and should feel good for both the giver and the receiver of the massage.

Through the giver's hula dance around the table and the flowing, energetic quality of the bodywork, energy is raised to assist in the removal of energy blocks in the receiver. Density in the receiver's body is softened through intent, compassion, love, and spirals of light through the giver's forearm. Lomi lomi can assist the receiver in re-experiencing her expanded self.

Lomi lomi is sometimes translated as "loving hands" massage and frequently may feel as though more than one person is performing the massage. The sharing of the breath, the essence of the Creator, or universal energy—whatever name you give it—is an old Hawaiian custom and greatly enhances the energy flow.

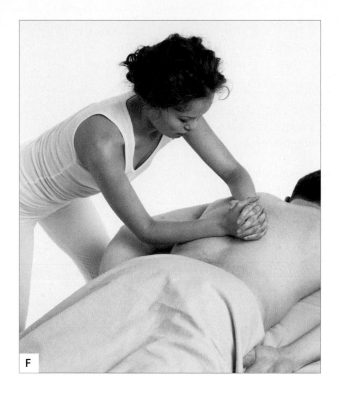

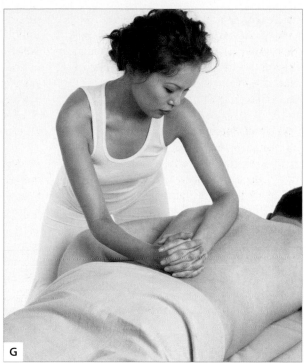

4. MASSAGE IN TWO PLACES WITH MANA LOI

Stand at the side of the table, facing your partner's hip, and clasp your fingers together. Your arms will make a V shape. Rolling them back and forth on your partner's back, hip, and shoulder areas in figure eights will give him the experience of having two areas massaged simultaneously. This technique, called mana loi, has the benefit of confusing tight muscles into relaxing because the receiver is unable to or can't hold his focus on more than one area of his body at a time. Meanwhile, you will be loosening your own back with the figure-eight movements of your torso (photos F and G).

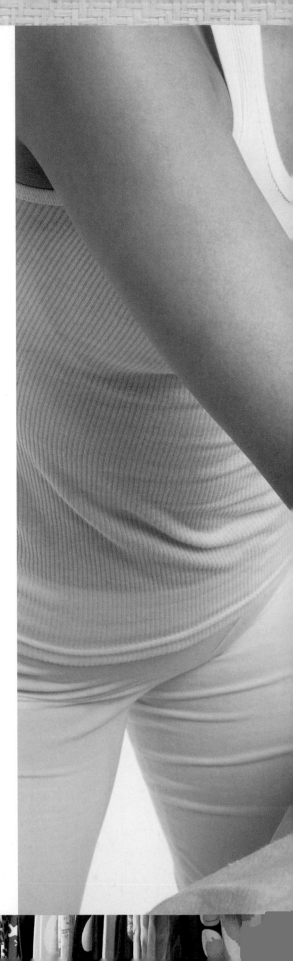

Circular Friction on the Sacrum

Hold the thumb of one of your hands in the fist of the other and make several figure eights around your partner's greater trochanter, the bone that is the most lateral in the hip area, until you feel some softening. This use of hands has a deeper effect than the forearms. Facing your partner's head, apply circular friction using your fingers or loose fists to sculpt just above the iliac crest as it arches from his sacrum out to his trochanter (**photo H**). You will feel vertical bands on the crest where the hardworking back muscles keep the spine erect; continue circles along the ilium until any ropey bands in the area become less apparent. Using your fingertips, apply small circular friction all over his sacrum to release any trapped energy held in the root of the spine and to invigorate the sacrum.

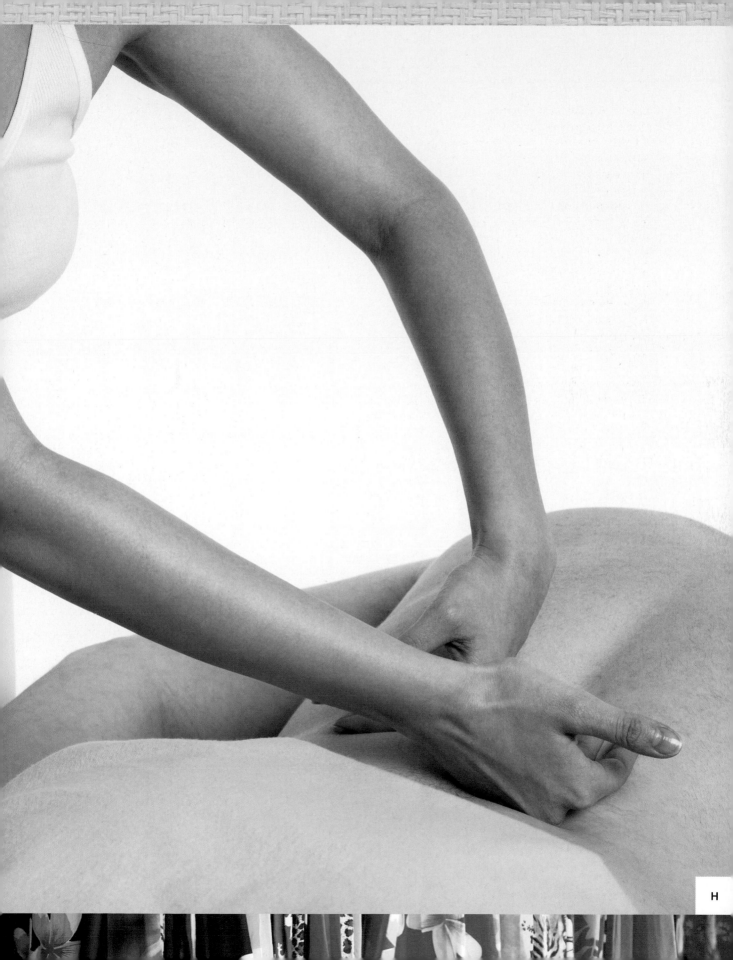

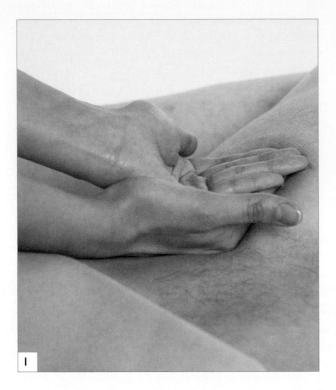

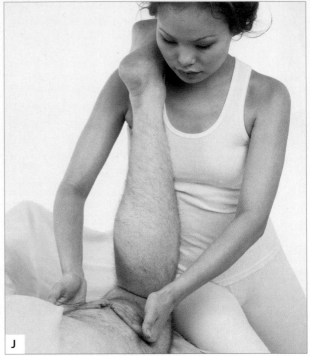

5. USE A GLACIALLY SLOW STROKE TO THE SHOULDER

Place your hands palms up, one supporting the other, and very slowly lean in and make a glacially slow, deep stroke toward your partner's shoulder **(photo I)**. The tissue moving ahead of your supported loose fist may be visualized as flowing lava. If at any point in this stroke you feel like the tissue is slowing or stopping your hands, give in to your intuition and hold your hands stationary in the spot until you feel the tissue loosen enough to allow you to continue with the moving stroke. Return to long gliding strokes, facing your partner's head, and glide with your right forearm perpendicular to his spine; make more circles and spirals with your forearm as you reach his shoulder.

6. PUT THE FOOT ON THE TABLE

Lift your partner's left foot, slowly pressing the front of his ankle forward, flexing his knee. Bring his foot only as close to his buttocks as the muscles freely allow. This puts a stretch on the quadriceps muscles of the anterior thigh, which can cause knee pain if they are chronically tight.

Lift the Leg and Mirror Circles

Sit on the table, just past your partner's left knee, and place his foot on your shoulder. With both hands in loose fists, make several mirror-image circles with your loose fists on his posterior thigh **(photo J)**, warming up the hamstring muscles. You may make a supported soft fist by placing one hand in the other palm and apply several strokes from above the back of his knee to the top of his thigh where it meets the buttock, gradually addressing the entire thigh.

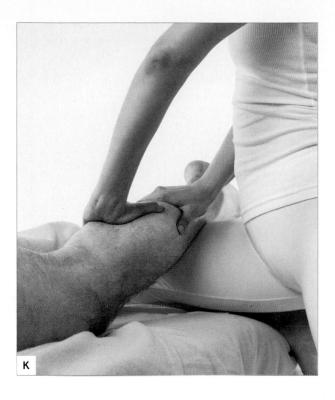

K

Warning!
Easy on the Calves

Ease into the calf muscles very gradually, especially if your partner is athletic, as these muscles can be very tight and tender.

Then use both hands to make large mirror-image circles on the medial and lateral thigh and calf muscles.

Wring the Calf Muscles and Stimulate the Sole

Hold your partner's lower leg up as you move to a standing position facing the table. Wring his calf vigorously, allowing his foot to move freely; then, holding the front of his ankle, use a loose fist to address the sole of his foot, flexing the ankle as you do so. You may also use a knuckle to spiral into the sole of the foot.

Knead and Roll the Calf Muscles

Still standing and facing the table, place your right knee on the table as you bring your partner's leg down toward it and place his ankle on your thigh **(photo K)**. Knead the calf muscles, endeavoring to make figure-eight-type movements as you pass the muscle tissue from one hand to the other, and be sure to keep your entire palm in contact with the muscle. Use a loose fist as you did on the thigh to address the length of the muscles from ankle to knee.

You may be able to perform some forearm rolling on the calf and thigh in this position if your back is flexible. Make several spiral strokes with a loose fist on the sole of your partner's foot, following the curve of his arch. You may use substantial pressure here. Take your knee off the table as you return your partner's foot to lie flat on its surface. If you have the length of reach to do so, you may cradle your partner's ankle on your forearm and move his leg as you work farther up his body. Loosening the calf muscles can help to prevent athletic or exertion injuries to the leg and ankle.

Lube Up!

This would be a good time to add some more oil to your hands before you turn and glide your forearm back down to your partner's foot.

7. GLIDE TO CREATE A CONNECTION, THEN ROCK AND ROLL THE SHOULDER AND ARM

Using your forearms, give your partner a feeling of connectedness on the entire left side of his body by gliding from his feet, up his legs and back, and down to his fingertips once or twice. If he is comfortable with the back of his wrist against the small of his back, you may place his arm there and put your left palm over his while you make circles with your fingers around the edge of his shoulder blade (scapula) **(photo L)**.

Then, with your hand underneath his, interlace your fingers with his and rotate his wrist before returning his arm to the table. Lift his left arm and carry it in front of you as you take a seat at the head of the table, with your right hip next to his armpit; then place his upper arm over your thigh. In this position, it is easy to knead the upper arm muscles, and you can roll his upper arm on your leg as you lean toward him and away from him a few times, broadening his shoulder each time you lean away. You may use your left forearm to spiral lightly into the triceps muscles on the back of his upper arm.

8. REPEAT THE SEQUENCE ON THE RIGHT

Come to the head of the table and use both forearms in spirals on your partner's back as a transition to the right side of his body. Repeat all the actions you performed on the left side and then return again to the head of the table. Starting at your partner's lower back, pull your arms, with palms facing up, toward you several times, alternating the strokes from your partner's low back to his shoulders. You are pulling energy back to the heart—both your partner's and your own—with a stroke called aloha lomi. Place your hands on his upper back for a few breaths before you have him turn over to a supine position.

History of Lomi Lomi

When the ancient Polynesians landed on the shores of Hawaii, they brought their traditional healing practices. Traditionally, lomi lomi was performed by kahunas, or shamans, who practiced the philosophy of Huna, although anyone and everyone could practice it in the island villages, from children to grandparents.

After American missionaries arrived in 1820 and converted many people on the islands to Christianity, traditional healing arts were prohibited and were dismissed as heathen and primitive. The complex healing system of lomi lomi, which included spiritual shamanic practices, herbal treatments, and the use of lava stones, went underground, but the restorative massage component remained popular among Hawaiians. In the 1970s, when the ban against traditional healing practices was lifted, Auntie Margaret Machado, a respected Hawaiian healer, and other traditional kahunas began bringing lomi lomi back into the public eye. This form of bodywork is now popular not just on the islands but around the world.

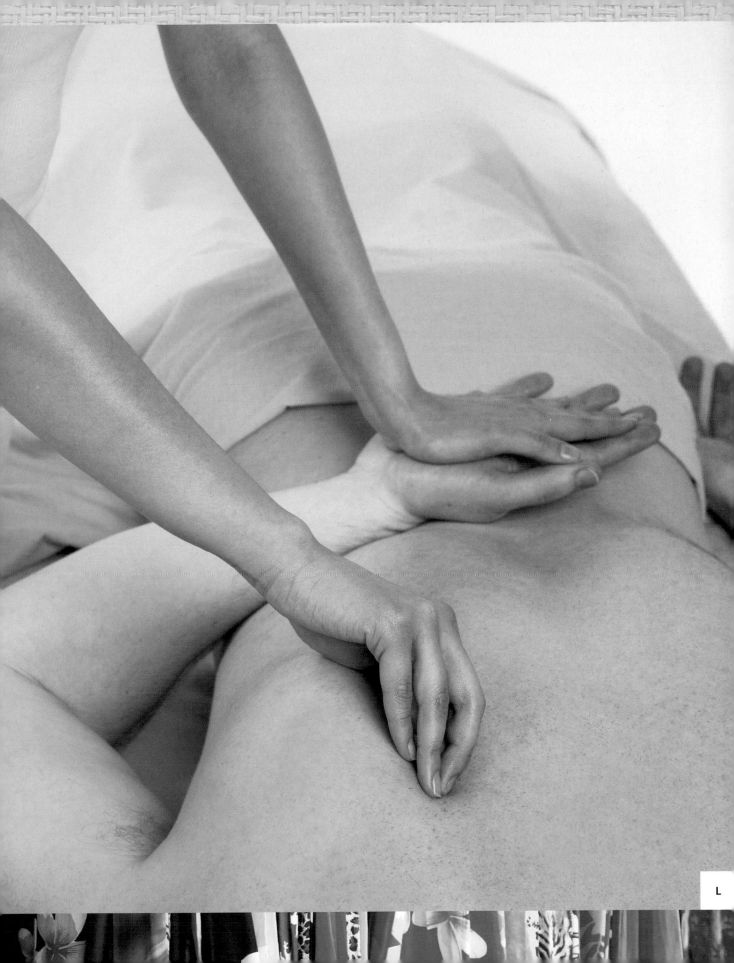

Lomi Lomi Supine Sequence

Much of the supine sequence of lomi lomi is focused on creating length in the neck, arm, and leg muscles and breadth in the chest and hip areas. Greater space in these areas created through fluid movements can feel very opening and freeing to the body, allowing for greater ease and grace of movement following the massage.

1. SUPPORT AND PULL THE NECK MUSCLES

Seated in a chair at the head of the table, hold your partner's head in your hands for a few breaths while you restore any wavering intention or focus. You will not need much oil on your hands for the neck massage, and too much may make it difficult to keep the pace of your strokes slow. Begin several alternating hand-pulling strokes from his shoulders, up his neck, and to the back of his head. Your hands should be cupped evenly around the back and sides of your partner's neck to ensure lengthening of as many of the neck muscles as possible. Keep the backs of your hands gliding over the surface of the table rather than lifting his head and lean back so that you put a gentle traction on his neck. The hand gliding up the back of his head should not release his head until your other hand is fully supporting and lengthening his neck; this will facilitate holding the head steady during the pulling strokes. After your last pull, let your hands meet and hold your partner's head. Rotate the back of his skull about 3 or 4 inches (7.6–10.2 cm) off the table, tucking his chin as you do so, and hold for one to three breaths. The pulling strokes and this neck stretch are very beneficial for lengthening the neck muscles, which become compressed and shortened from carrying the weight of the head and which are prime repositories for day-to-day tension.

Circular Friction on the Occipital Ridge

Placing your partner's head back on the table, curve your fingers and use your fingertips to make small circles along the occipital ridge, or base of the skull, back and forth from his spine to the bump below his ear (the mastoid process). Move back and forth along the ridge a few times to loosen the attachments of several muscles, feeling for areas of tension where you might pause and hold stationary compression. Apply the same circular friction strokes parallel to his spine, from the base of his skull down to his lower neck and back up to his occiput. Repeat at least three times, moving laterally a bit with each pass. Then, starting at the base of his neck, with your fingers to each side of his spine, lift your fingers skyward, then toward you, moving a little farther up with each ocean wave-type stroke (i.e., a "come here" motion). When your fingers arrive at the occiput, passively stretch your partner's neck by leaning back and holding for a few breaths. Release the hold slowly on your partner's exhalation.

For Ease, Stand While Pulling the Neck

If your partner's head is very heavy or if you lack the muscular strength to perform this stroke while seated, stand with your knees and hips flexed and your thighs supported against the head of the table to rise into a position that may offer you more mechanical advantage. If you use this stance, lean back into your hips for stability and to create traction on the neck.

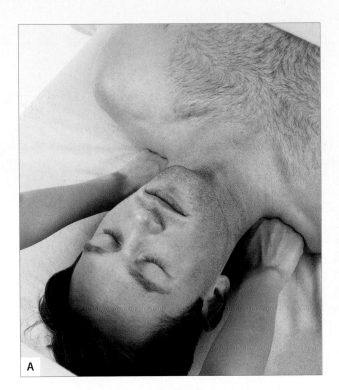

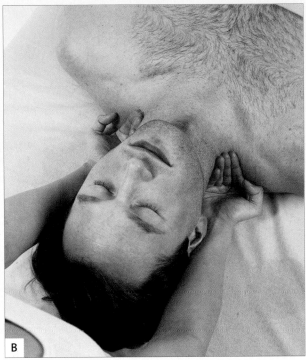

2. USE FIGURE EIGHTS ON THE NECK AND UPPER SHOULDERS

With the backs of the fingers of both hands against the lateral back of your partner's neck, glide down to his shoulders **(photo A)**. Rotate your wrists outward so that your fingers are pointing skyward for their return back up to the base of his skull **(photo B)**. When your hands are almost to the mastoid processes, rotate your wrists inward and glide back down his neck again with your fingers pointing toward the table surface. Keep the movements fluid and your hands soft. You may continue this figure-eight movement on his neck until you feel that he has released any holding of his head and neck. A variation is to turn his head to the left, holding at the occiput with your left hand to lengthen his neck, and do the figure-eight strokes only with your right hand, which will allow you to go a little farther into his shoulder on the right side. Repeat on his left side.

Circle across the Upper Chest

Standing at the left side of the table near your partner's shoulder, use your right hand in a soft fist to lean in with circles across his pectoralis, or upper chest muscles, while you hold under his left scapula with your left hand, fingertips curved around the medial edge of the bone. You may go all the way across his chest, making sure to lighten up as you pass over his sternum, and make circles all the way back over to his left shoulder. Placing your right hand with your palm firmly down on his left shoulder and keeping your left hand under it, rotate the shoulder as you hold it between your palms.

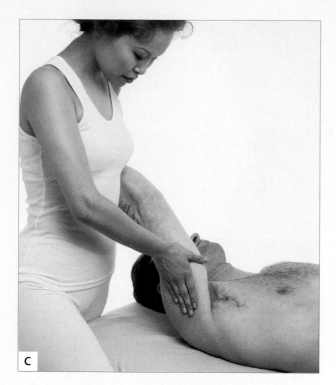

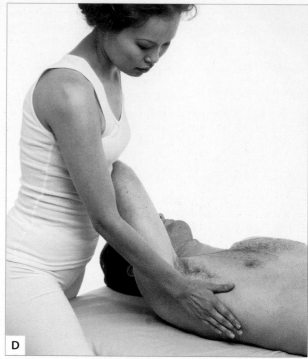

3. GLIDE FROM THE FOREARM TO THE WAIST

Take your partner's left hand in yours and lean back as you bring his arm perpendicular to his chest or overhead for his **(photo C)**. Keeping length in the arm, use your palm to glide from your partner's forearm to his upper arm, then down the side of his chest to his waist **(photo D)**. If he is much taller than you are, you may need to hold his forearm against your body with your arm to make the length of the stroke to his waist. Then, standing at the head of the table, hold his forearm on your right forearm with his elbow flexed so that his elbow is almost directly over his shoulder. Knead the back of his upper arm (the triceps muscle) firmly with your full left palm, adding some circular movements with both the working hand and your right arm. This will help to confuse the muscle into relaxing and letting go. Return his arm to the table and make a few gliding connecting strokes from fingertips to shoulders and back with your left hand as you hold his right hand in your own. Repeat the chest and arm movements on the right side of his body. Much of the discomfort felt in the upper back is from tight chest and anterior shoulder muscles, so massaging these areas has benefits on both the front and back upper torso.

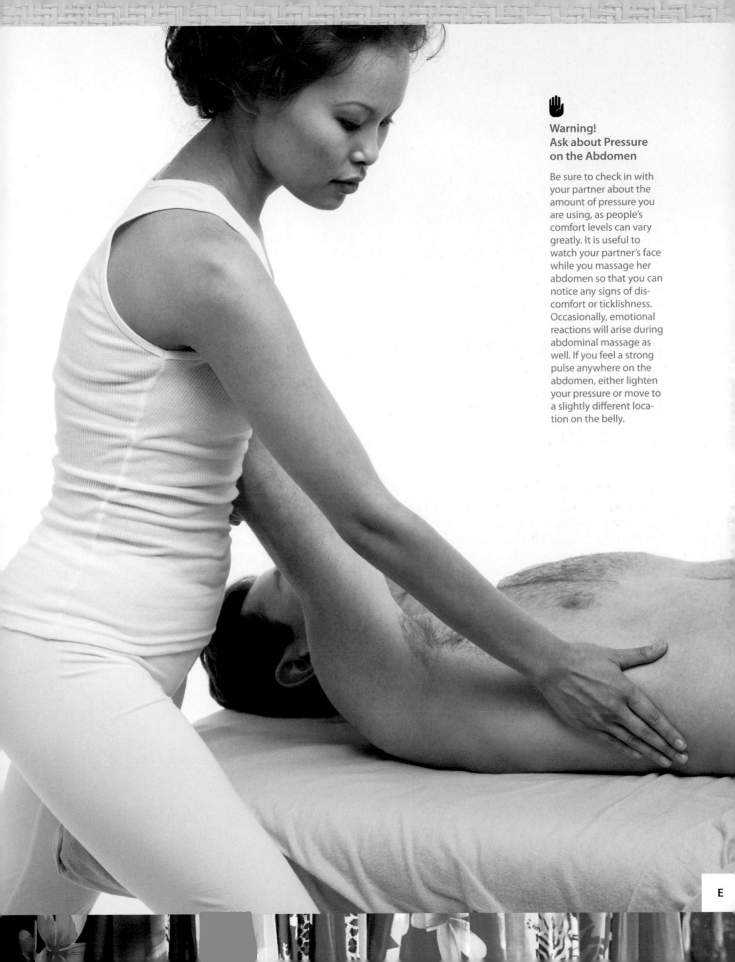

Warning!
**Ask about Pressure
on the Abdomen**

Be sure to check in with
your partner about the
amount of pressure you
are using, as people's
comfort levels can vary
greatly. It is useful to
watch your partner's face
while you massage her
abdomen so that you can
notice any signs of dis-
comfort or ticklishness.
Occasionally, emotional
reactions will arise during
abdominal massage as
well. If you feel a strong
pulse anywhere on the
abdomen, either lighten
your pressure or move to
a slightly different location on the belly.

4. PLACE YOUR HANDS ON THE ABDOMEN

Remaining on the right side of the table and facing toward the head, bring your hands slowly onto your partner's abdomen and hold one hand above the navel and one below it for two or three breaths. This is an energetically sensitive part of the body, so all of your movements should be slow, conscious, and deliberate.

Clockwise Circles on the Abdomen

Begin moving your hands gently in clockwise circles to spread oil on your partner's abdomen. One hand moves in a full circle, and the other forms a crescent as it moves in the same direction to give the feeling of continuous circles around the navel. Then place one hand over the other and continue a little more firmly, but not leaning in heavily, in clockwise circles between his lower rib cage and his lower pelvis for a few circles. Locate the intersection of his lower ribs above his belly; this is the zyphoid process of the sternum and it marks the starting point for three light strokes down to the navel.

Deepen the Move to Improve Digestion

Either have your partner place his feet flat on the table with his knees elevated or place a cushion or two under his knees before you work more deeply. Next, have him inhale deeply and then exhale completely. When all the air is expelled, perform the stroke again, a little more deeply, from the zyphoid process to the navel, on one of your exhalations, relatively quickly. Repeat this move three times. It is thought to have the effect of creating a bit of a vacuum to facilitate movement of the contents of the stomach and upper gastrointestinal tract into the intestines.

Rock the Side with Ocean Waves

Reach across your partner's torso near his waistline and scoop the tissue toward you, using your right hand and forearm at the same time as you push from his side waist closest to you with your left hand and forearm. Your forearms will pass each other as you move them in opposite directions in ocean-wave strokes (photos F and G). Rock forward and back and let the movement come from your whole body rather than just making the movement with your arms. Using both hands and forearms, reach further under the opposite side of your partner's back, pulling toward yourself with one hand, then the other, alternating as you move up and down his side from hip to armpit. Don't pass the midline as you perform these raking strokes but stop at the navel. Curl your fingers slightly and try to follow the indentations between the ribs if you can feel them. If your arms are long enough, you may reach under both sides of your partner's back almost to the vertebral column at the waistline and pull both hands simultaneously around his sides and to the navel. Do this bilateral pulling stroke once or twice. All of these strokes have the effect of loosening the lower back by lifting it and enhancing the forward lumbar curve of the spine.

Finish Abdominal Massage with Vibration

Finish massaging the abdomen with a few very light counterclockwise circles followed by a somewhat deeper clockwise one; then place your hand over your partner's navel and vibrate your hand for several seconds, with the vibration coming from your shoulder. Allow your hand to lie still on your partner's abdomen for a few breaths and then move to the side of the table by your partner's right leg.

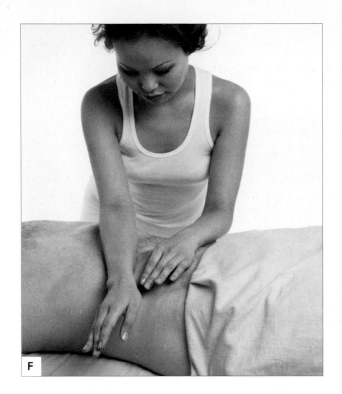

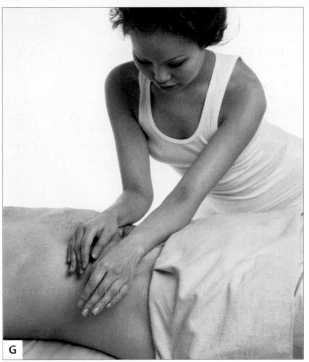

The Abdomen's Important Role

Hawaiians traditionally have used the same word for the large intestine as is used for the emotional heart or soul, and in the philosophy of Huna, the abdomen is considered a very important part of the body to massage. Lomi lomi abdominal massage is called opu huli.

5. LUBRICATE THE LEG FROM THE TOES TO THE HIP

Place an abundant amount of oil into your palms and blow into them. Spread the oil from your partner's toes up to his hips, being sure to get the medial and lateral surfaces of his leg and thigh. Many people have dry skin on their legs, so it may take more oil than you expect (and men with hairy legs require even more oil so that the hair doesn't feel pulled). Spiral one of your forearms, then both forearms, up his thigh relatively lightly (**photo H**). Clasp your hands and make several figure eights up and down his thigh from the side, gradually sinking your body weight into the strokes more deeply. Warm the tissue with ocean waves, pulling the medial thigh toward you as you push the lateral thigh tissue away from you, with your hands passing each other as they move back and forth across the thigh, gradually working up toward the hip and down to the knee.

Circle around the Knee

Holding your hands as though you are cupping a bowl, make circles around your partner's knee with the ulnar sides of your hands. The circular motion should come from turning your entire body rather than just your hands. This movement relaxes the muscles and ligaments that cross the front of the knee joint, helping to keep the muscles balanced and the knee tracking properly.

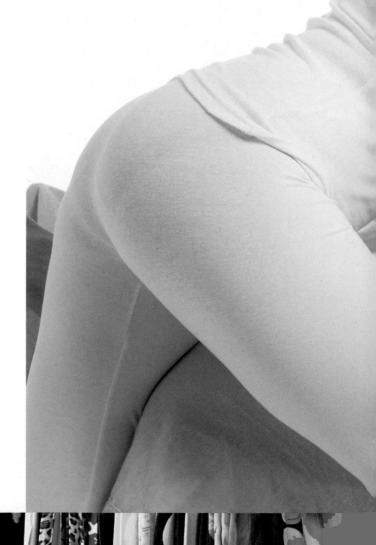

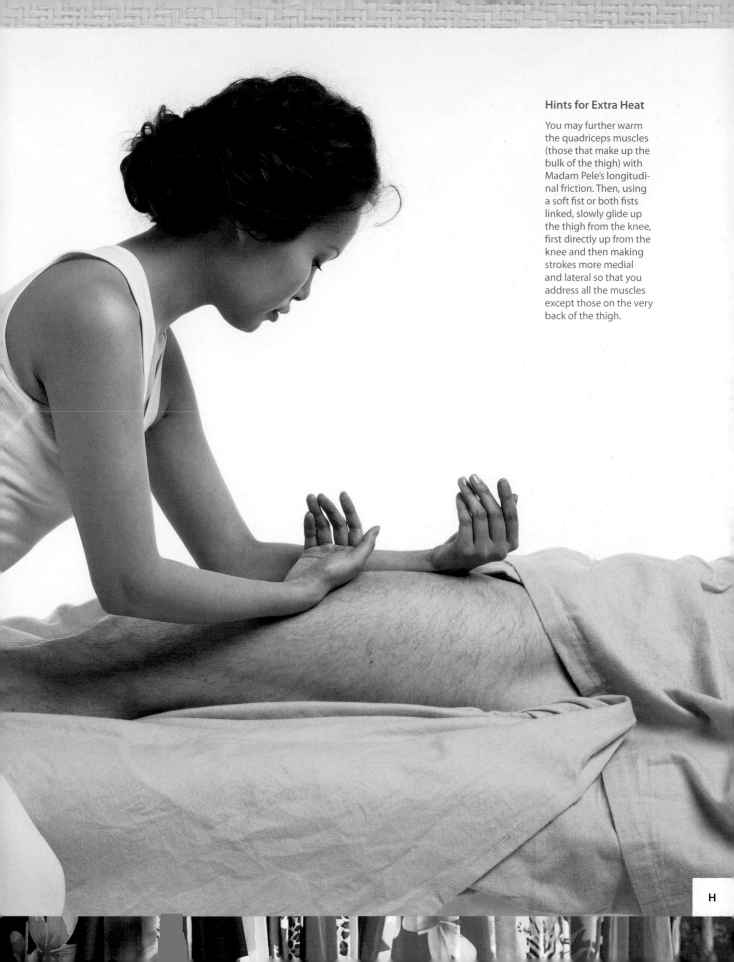

Hints for Extra Heat

You may further warm the quadriceps muscles (those that make up the bulk of the thigh) with Madam Pele's longitudinal friction. Then, using a soft fist or both fists linked, slowly glide up the thigh from the knee, first directly up from the knee and then making strokes more medial and lateral so that you address all the muscles except those on the very back of the thigh.

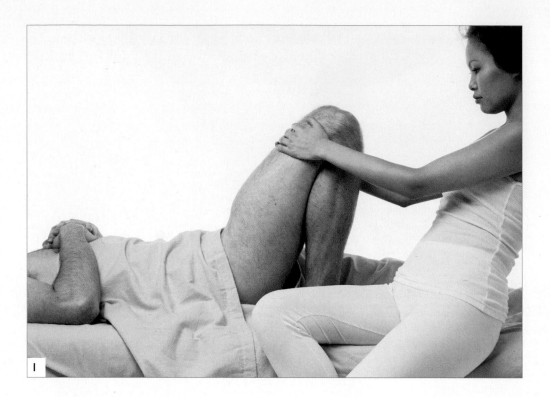

I

Use a Rocking Rhythm to Loosen the Thigh

Lift your partner's knee up as you press the sole of his foot toward his hip, placing the sole flat on the table. Take a seat just past his toes and wrap your arms around his thighs; then lean back and hold the thigh in a comfortable stretch. Begin rocking forward and back and side to side while holding his thigh, finding his natural rhythm **(photo I)**. You do not need to push the limb away from you, but simply lean your body weight back in different positions and find out how quickly his body recoils when you release the pressure. This rhythmic rocking assists in loosening the low back, thigh, and groin muscles. As you perform these range-of-motion actions, your partner's leg will gradually move farther than its initial movement allowed. Continue until you feel you have reached your partner's comfortable range-of-motion limitation.

Work the Inner Thigh

Stand with your left knee just past your partner's toes and encourage his leg and thigh to rotate out to the side. Have a pillow or your knee available to support his knee if his leg and thigh do not drop naturally to the surface of the table. Spiral lightly with your left forearm, from his knee up toward his groin, working sensitively as the inner thigh can be tender **(photo J)**. You may use a soft fist to further address the inner thigh muscles (the adductors) from the knee upward.

Chronically held tension in the adductor muscles actually can contribute to hip tightness and discomfort, so creating length in these inner thigh muscles can help release discomfort in the lateral and posterior hips.

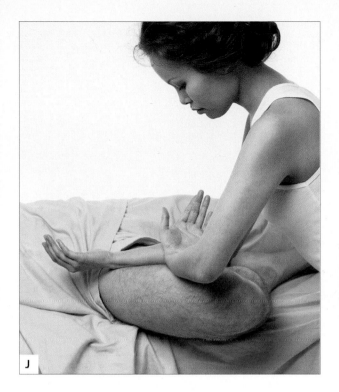

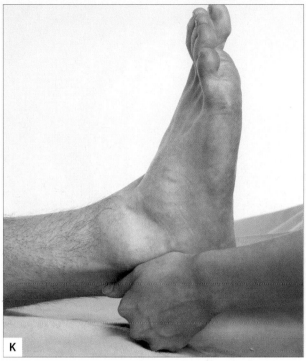

Spread and Circle from the Knees to the Heels

Bring your partner's knee back up toward the sky and extend his leg, creating some traction at his hip joint by holding his upper calf with both hands underneath it, palms upward. Starting just below his knee, spread the muscles toward your palms using your thumbs and thumb pads (thenar eminences), moving away from his shin. Repeat these spreading strokes all the way down his leg.

Use your fingertips to apply circular friction within his comfort level with the pressure to the medial and lateral calf muscles as you work your way back up his leg to his knee and return to his foot. On his heel, just below his ankle bones, apply circular friction with either your fingertips or your thenar eminences (**photo K**). The heels have connections to the uterus, and using circular friction on women's heels may assist in relieving menstrual cramps; plus, it just feels good to have an area stimulated that we seldom think about.

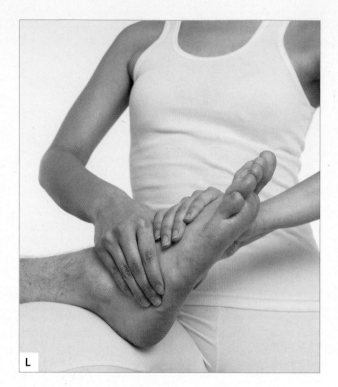

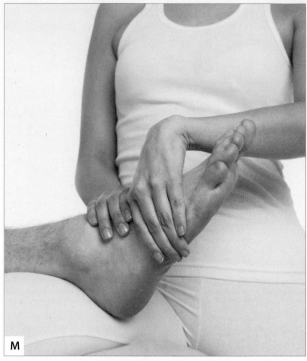

6. WRING THE FOOT AND CONNECT WITH LONG STROKES

Sit on the side of the table and place your partner's foot on your thigh. In this position, you can easily rotate his ankle and perform wringing motions on his foot with your hands moving in opposite directions, stimulating the arches of the foot **(photos L, M, and N)**. With the Achilles tendon area on the top of your thigh, you can press on his forefoot and lean toward the end of the table, putting a nice traction on his entire leg. Lift his leg and return to a standing position at the side of the table; then connect the limb from toes to groin with a few gliding strokes.

7. REPEAT THE SEQUENCE ON THE OTHER SIDE

Move to the opposite side of the table and massage your partner's other leg, thigh, and foot. Finish by coming to the head of the table and placing both hands on his head or upper chest or place one hand on his head or chest and raise the other to channel energy. Maintain the same kind of prayerful attitude with which you started the session for several breaths before you break contact.

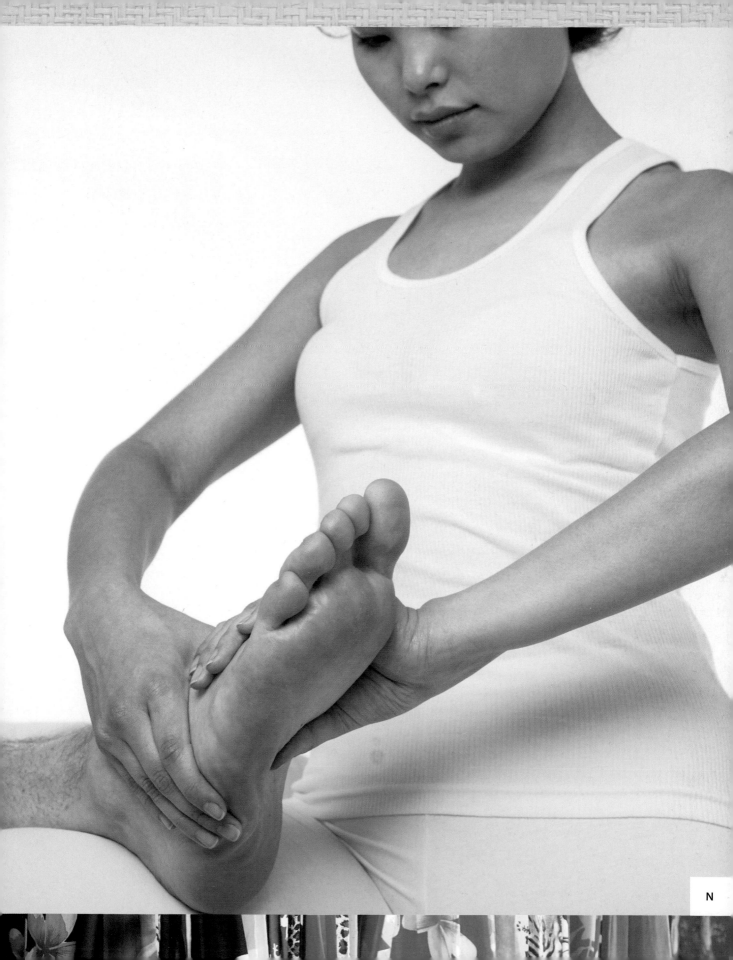

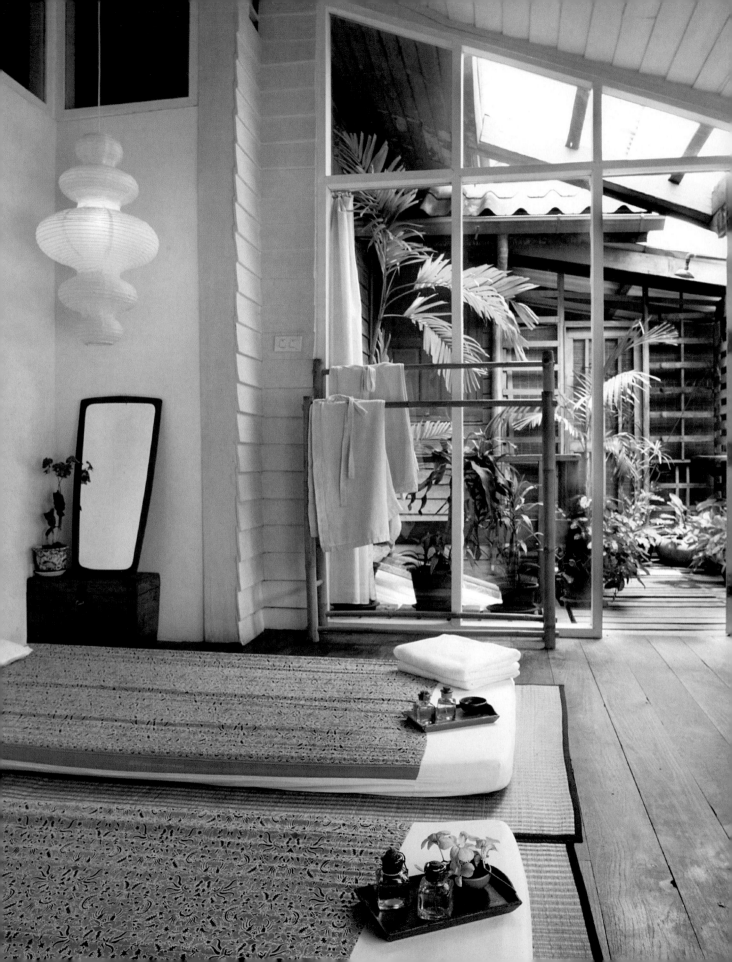

CHAPTER 6

Tantsu Enfolds and Supports the Receiver

All of the bodywork modalities in this book are suitable for sharing with your partner, children, parents, and friends—except possibly this form. Harold Dull, the wonderfully poetic originator of Watsu, an aquatic bodywork based on Zen shiatsu (detailed in chapter 8), created Tantsu by bringing Watsu back out of the water and onto the mat. The water in Watsu surrounds and supports the receiver, and the giver mostly "disappears," being the same temperature as the water. In Tantsu, the comforting, interconnected support you provide for your partner is based on close cradling and enfolding.

Tantsu focuses on sensing and responding to what you discover in your partner and allowing a more naturally healthy state to emerge. You are inviting your partner's body to express itself within the safety of your supportive holding, and in this safe space, your responses to what you feel may lead you to knead, stretch, stroke, or apply pressure as your partner's body instructs. Your partner's body leads the dance. This is massage as co-creation—focused play.

How Intimate Is It?

As a Watsu practitioner, I hold people I barely know in my arms in the water and put them through stretches with close body contact, and it doesn't seem to make them (or me!) uncomfortable. Although I am especially open to all varieties of bodywork and close contact, I think some people might be a bit uncomfortable giving a Tantsu session in the anterior position to someone other than an intimate partner. As noted in the text, a Tantsu session can be done with your partner lying on either side and facing away from you rather than moving into a position facing you, and most people are comfortable with the level of intimacy in that position. Indeed, one of the lovely things about Tantsu is how comfortable being cradled in the side-lying position is for most people. Tantsu fosters resonance between two individuals and a deep letting go into focused, supportive nurturing.

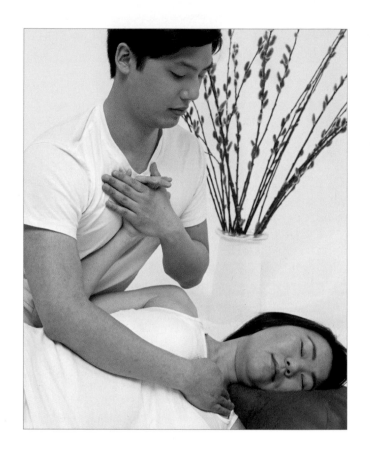

Tantsu Strokes and Pressure Guidelines

- Forearm rolls and lifts are executed with just enough pressure to gently move the tissue to its normal limit in range of motion, just as with gentle pulling and pushing with hands.
- Thumbing areas for deeper effect should be performed slowly and consciously, progressively sinking in until meeting resistance from the tissues.
- Holding hands on the heart is tender and nurturing, like a mother's hand on a sick child's forehead.
- Compression releases tension, but ease in slowly and only as far as the tissue seems to invite you to come.

Pre-Tantsu Breathing Exercise

Most of us don't notice the global quality of our breath in our bodies. This is an exercise to get you in touch with your breath so that you may better use it in Tantsu. Lie on your back, with your knees supported by a cushion for comfort. Allow your breath to deepen, really drawing air into your belly as well as your lungs. As you breathe, start noticing how your chest expands and your shoulders elevate toward your ears with each inhalation, easing back down on the exhalations. Notice the opening of your chest on the inhalations and how your relaxed arms will rotate outward slightly on inhalations and roll inward on exhalations. Allow your attention to move downward to your belly and hips, feeling how your abdomen rises and your hip bones flare outward on the inhalations, and then to your legs, which will also tend to roll outward on each inhalation. You may feel an overall expansion throughout your body on inhalations and a subsiding or contraction in all your tissues on the exhalations. It is interesting to note that another word for inhalation is inspiration. Your partner's breath informs and inspires your movements, from the beginning to the end of the session.

Preparation for Tantsu

- Any exercise like yoga or meditation to still your mind and focus may be useful before a session. Coordinating breath and movement in your yoga practice will prepare you especially well for a Tantsu session.
- Be dressed in loose, comfortable clothing, with bare feet, and have your partner do the same.
- You'll need a firm mat, a meditation pillow, or a folded blanket or towel, and three cushions.
- Be sure your partner knows that you will respond to any feedback about her comfort immediately, and that she should make sure to shift her position to enhance comfort whenever necessary.

Tantsu Posterior Hold Sequence

These instructions will give you a starting point—a sense for how a session may unfold—but the essence of Tantsu is to be in the moment, responding to whatever movement or stillness arises in your partner rather than performing a fixed sequence. As long as your intention is to assist your partner in whatever unfolding will be beneficial for her body and you are fully present in your heart as well as your arms, your session will be filled with openness and trust.

1. GET CLOSE AND COMFORTABLE ON THE FLOOR

To begin, sit on the cushion and have your partner lie comfortably on her left side in a fetal position, in front of you with her back to you. Your left foot should be tucked between yourself and your partner, with your thigh behind her occiput, unless it is uncomfortable. Other options include flexing your left leg as though kneeling or extending it under the cushion supporting her head. Your right knee will be at her hip, supported with a pillow or a folded blanket. Make sure you're in a comfortable position, even if you have to adjust your legs in other ways. Add cushions anywhere else they will add to your partner's comfort and your own.

2. LENGTHEN WITH THE FOREARMS AND BREATH

Place your relaxed left forearm above your partner's shoulder and your right forearm below her hip with just enough pressure so that her inhalations will slightly push your forearms apart, encouraging your chest to open, drawing back in with the exhalations. Sink into the rhythm of your partner's breath. At the end of each shared exhalation, let the emerging in-breath push your arms apart and draw you up, through your heart space and extending out through your arms. Until you feel some intuitive direction from your partner's body and breath, just allow your arms to move effortlessly in and out with the breath. Usually one arm will feel the influence of your partner's breath more than the other, and this gives you the first direction to lead into movement.

Forearm Rolling on the Lower Back and Hip

When it feels right, allow your partner's forearm to move around her hip area, then from her hip to her lower back, and maintain stillness for a few breaths. Then sink in, rock forward, or make other movements your forearm is drawn into **(photo A)**. To use your forearms, you must move your body more from your core than your hands. Your left forearm maintains contact with the breath while the other explores what the breath is doing in the hip and back by slowly rolling in both areas. Gradually allow your right shoulder to move more in rotation. The more you use your shoulder, the more your whole body will be engaged in the dance that unfolds.

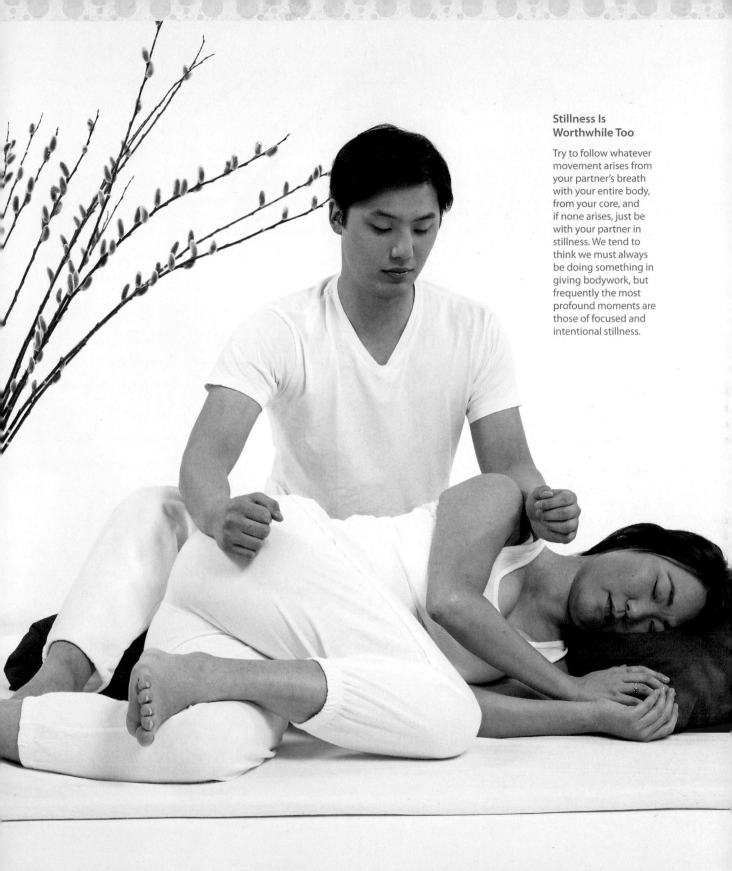

Try to follow whatever
movement arises from
your partner's breath
with your entire body,
from your core, and
if none arises, just be
with your partner in
stillness. We tend to
think we must always
be doing something in
giving bodywork, but
frequently the most
profound moments are
those of focused and
intentional stillness.

A

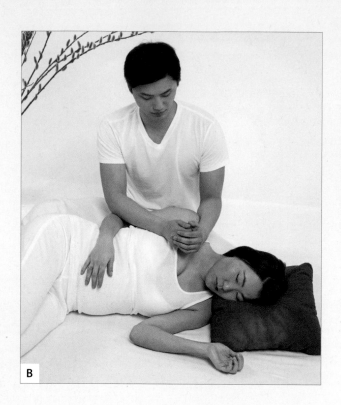

B

Release Displaced Tension

Often the restrictions we feel in our lower backs actually come from more lateral muscles, especially near the waist, and this stretch will create more flexibility and ease in the whole back. The same is true near the shoulder, where several muscles can shorten the side of the back behind the armpit, limiting range of motion in the shoulder, which this sequence can improve. Place your partner's hand behind her head and rotate her elbow, especially moving it forward and back, into different positions. Avoid this part of the sequence if she has a history of shoulder dislocations.

3. ROTATE THE SHOULDER AND STRETCH THE NECK

As you feel drawn up into the upper body, bring your right forearm up toward the back of your partner's shoulder and clasp her shoulder between your forearms, lifting and rotating it in whatever ways you feel drawn to explore (**photo B**). You will notice that rotations not only gradually increase the range of motion in her shoulder; they will also lengthen and stretch the side of her neck, which is often tight. That tightness can contribute to pain, numbness, weakness, and tingling in the forearms and hands and fluid range-of-motion movements may help relieve those symptoms.

Twist the Torso

Reach under your partner's arm with your right forearm; then lay her arm back over your thigh. Lean into her chest just medial to the deltoid with your left forearm and into the lower back with your right forearm. Stretch her lower back while keeping her chest open by pulling with your left forearm; find a point of balance in the core of your body. This will put a gentle twist into her torso. Begin to explore alternating pressure with each of your forearms, allowing your shoulders to move freely and enhancing mobility in her torso.

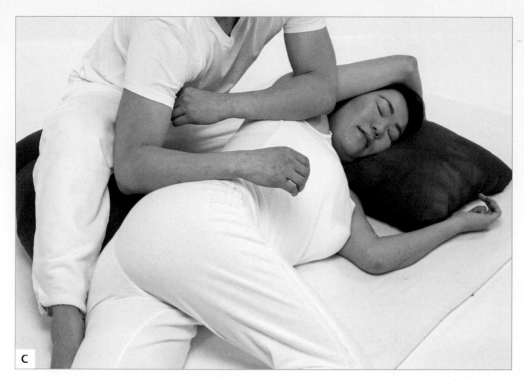

C

Warning!
Be Aware of Previous
Shoulder Injury

It may be best to leave
out shoulder rotations
if your partner has any
history of shoulder
dislocations.

Thumb along the Shoulder Blade

You may bring your right hand behind your
partner's back and press with your thumb along
the medial border of her scapula (shoulder
blade) as you use your left forearm to create
backward pressure onto your thumb, but only
do so if it is not a strain on your wrist. Pulling her
shoulder back onto your thumb has a less inva-
sive feel to it than pressing in strongly with your
thumb, and your partner may be able to relax
into it more. This area is prone to ropy muscles
and knots, and releasing them can help alleviate
upper back discomfort. By bringing awareness
and openness into the heart area, her posture
may gradually improve as well.

Push and Pull to Open the Body

Allow your forearm to move back to your partner's hip and continue pushing forward with it
while you pull back to open her chest. This takes
the stretch farther down in her body, opening
her hips as well. This push/pull has a balancing
and opening effect on the body **(photo C)**.

4. HOLD THE HEART AND HEAD STILL

Holding the heart area open with your left forearm, place your right hand on your partner's
heart center. Breathe together to connect in
stillness for as long as your intuition tells you.
Release her shoulder and place your left hand
on her cheek, making a connection between
heart and head. Keep your hands in the two
positions for a few breaths and then place
your left hand farther back, on her temple, and
hold for a few breaths. Repeat with the heel of
your hand at the base of her skull, holding and
breathing. Your right hand remains on her heart
center as you move your left hand to the different positions on her head.

Keep a Posture of Openness

Be sure to keep your
chest, hereafter called
your heart, open; avoid
rounding your shoulders
or dropping your head
and neck forward. You
will avoid discomfort by
keeping your shoulders
low and broad and main-
taining openness in the
front of your torso, much
like the openness you
are encouraging in your
partner's chest.

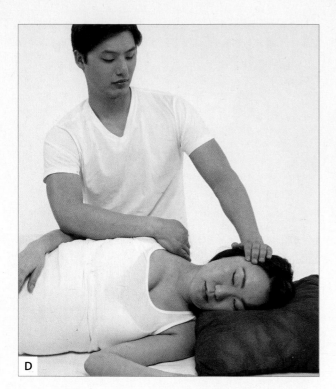

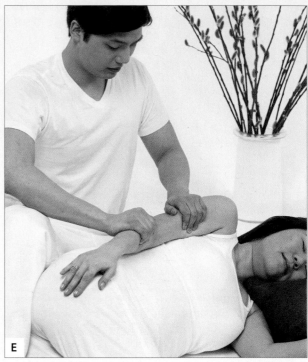

Stretch the Neck

Move your right hand from your partner's heart center to her shoulder, exerting a gentle downward pull, stretching her neck **(photo D)**. This position, which you hold in stillness, keeping some dynamic tension in the stretch, adds to the hand, arm, and neck benefits of the shoulder rotations performed earlier in the sequence. Further loosening of the lateral neck may be realized by pressing several points with the palm of your left hand, working down toward the shoulder.

Repeat the Shoulder Rotations

Rotate your partner's shoulder, using a hand on each side of it, as you did with your forearms, gradually opening into larger circles as the shoulder loosens. The direction of the rotation is not critical, but moving her shoulder in the direction it would take if she were sweeping her hair back from her face will have more ben-

efit for shortened chest muscles. If she seems to be either guarding or assisting you in the shoulder rotations, make some random reversals in direction to perhaps confuse her into passively receiving the range of motion. Do not be concerned about popping or creaking noises coming from your partner's shoulder unless she expresses discomfort with the movement.

Squeeze and Lift the Arm

Place your partner's hand and arm along her side. Holding her upper arm with your left hand, press downward on your exhalations as though you are squeezing the air out of her arm, moving down her arm toward her wrist **(photo E)**. When you reach her wrist, lift her arm on an inhalation. Feel the weight and relaxation in the arm you are holding and explore movement with her arm, possibly holding it against your belly or your shoulder and leaning back for a stretch.

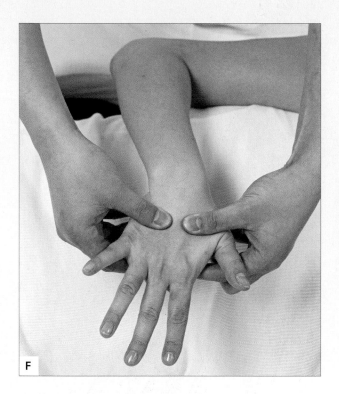

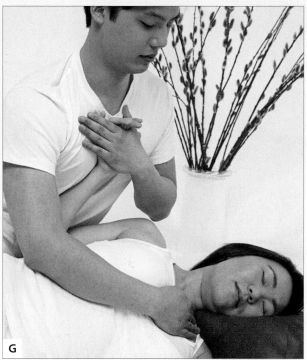

Make the Hand/Heart Connection

Hold your partner's hand in both of your own. Explore opening and spreading her palm, closing it upon itself and gently rotating her wrist (**photo F**). Place the back of her hand against your own heart with your right hand, reaching with your left arm in front of her shoulder, and place her hand on her heart, sinking into the breath together (**photo G**). Bring her arm overhead and then bring her upper arm over her ear and cross your arms so that your left hand works down her side to her hip and your right hand encourages length in her arm. Direct your weight not straight down into the muscles but at an angle to further the stretches in whatever way her body invites. Using your right hand, place her hand behind her on your right thigh or in front of her with her hand resting on the mat.

Fine-motor Freedom

Releasing tension from the arm and hand can help prevent or improve tightness and repetitive strain from computer use or other hand-intensive work.

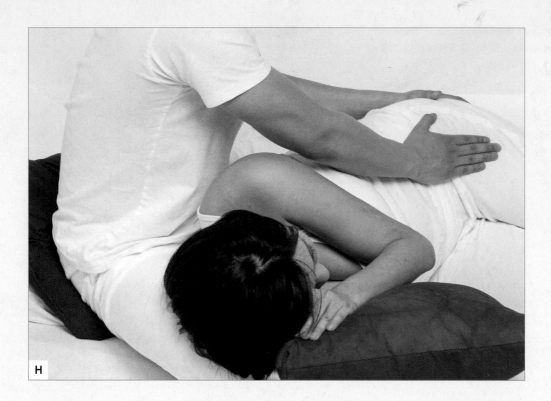

H

5. CONTAIN AND ROCK THE HARA

Place your hand on your partner's abdomen, right below the navel (called the hara), with your other hand on her heart center for several breaths. Then take your hand from her heart center and place it on the hara as you remove your right hand and place it directly behind the hara on her lower back **(photo H)**. Contain the hara between your hands, and if you feel called to do so, rock the area forward and backward a few times. This can release chronically held emotional tension from the belly and relieve the various gastrointestinal difficulties which are exacerbated by stress. It can also aid in digestion and stimulate free movement of energy through this pivotal energetic center of the body.

Explore the Hip, Leg, and Ankle

Keep your left hand on your partner's hara and explore the area around the hip joint and buttock with compressions and rocking **(photo I)**. Use your thumb to press into the indentations on and around the sacrum. Then hold the hip between your hands and roll it forward and back, gradually slowing into stillness. Follow this by holding at the hip with your left hand and applying compressions with your hand or forearm all the way down your partner's leg.

Hold her lower leg in both hands and lean back to a point of comfortable balance. Let her leg suggest to you what rotations and movements will be beneficial. Consider placing your partner's foot on the mat in front of her and pull her knee back toward you using both hands. You may find yourself led to rock her knee toward her head gently to moderate tightness in her hip and lower back. If her flexibility allows for it, bring her arm behind your body. With your hands curved so that your entire palm and fingers are in contact with her thigh, perform squeezing compressions, or kneading, all along both the front and back of her thigh and down her leg into her calf muscles.

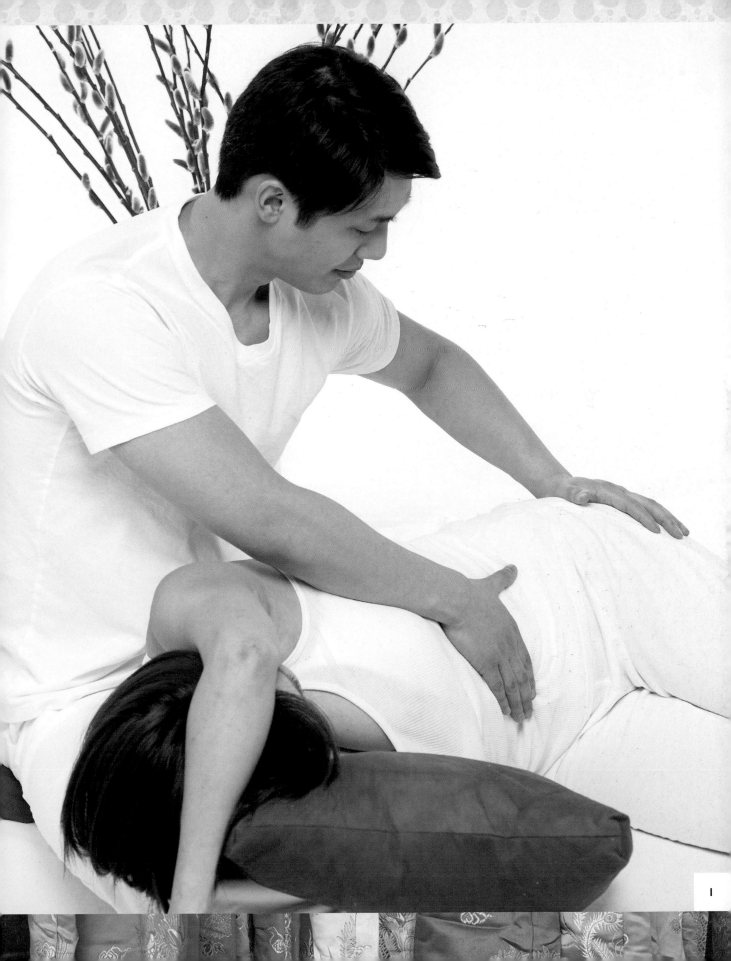

Enjoy a Synovial Bath

You might bring your partner's knee toward her shoulder, with her lower leg in line with her thigh, and again pull back toward you with both hands **(photo J)**. This position sets up the possibility of placing your right hand under her calf and rotating her leg or lifting her ankle with your left hand while using your right hand or forearm to press along the back of her thigh. Before you release her leg back down, you may want to explore her foot, stretching and compressing it like you did for her hand, rotating the ankle, opening and closing the sole of the foot, and wringing it. These moves can increase mobility in hip, knee, and ankle joints, contributing to a smoother and more graceful gait and decreasing stiffness by bathing the joints in synovial fluid.

Being in Tune

Just as tuning forks vibrate together when a note is struck on one fork, numerous studies have demonstrated that individuals' nervous systems synchronize when they are close to one another. Tantsu enhances this enmeshment for profound relaxation and change. The receiver's body invites the giver to enter into a flow, which re-educates the body's habitual reactions. Ideally, the giver is in a moving meditation, staying fully present and interactive with whatever is found in the receiver's body, allowing new restorative patterns to arise.

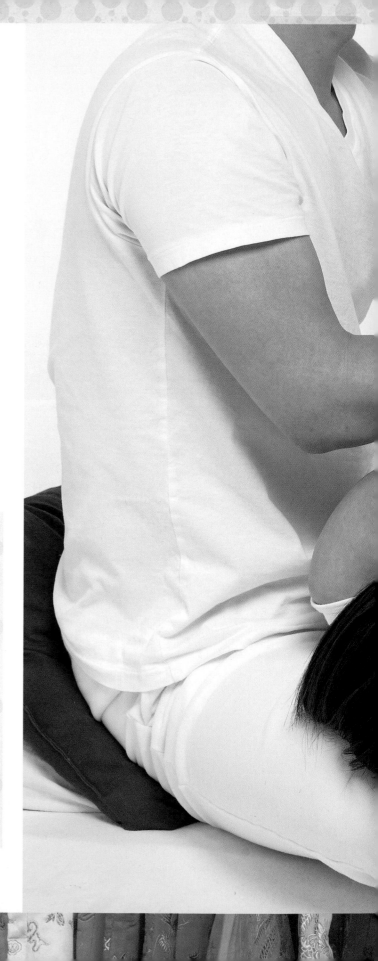

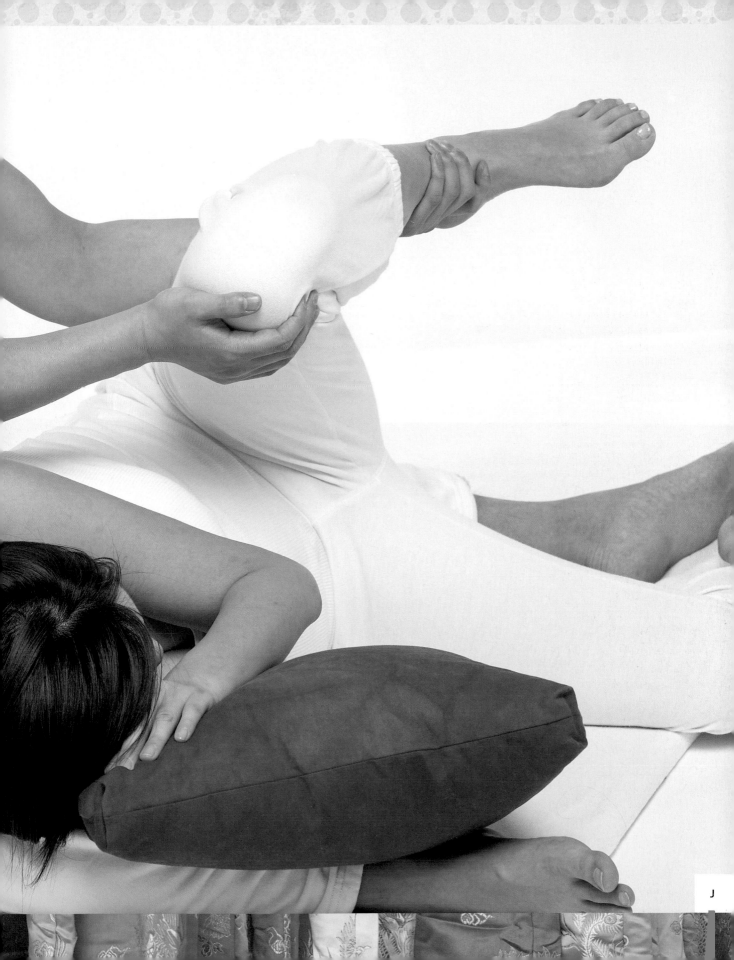

6. RETURN YOUR PARTNER TO A FETAL POSITION

Take your partner's leg onto the mat and carefully flex her knee and rotate her ankle, work foot points (see page 108), wring her foot, and then put it down, with the sole of her foot against your own sole. With your partner once again settled into a fetal position, place your hands on her hara and heart and hold for several breaths. You may want to lean your head and chest on your partner's hip and thigh as you relax your arms to cradle her legs or find another enveloping position that is comfortable for you both to use as a pause or as an ending. This is a point at which you might consider stopping if time is limited. Although you will have worked primarily one side of your partner's body, the other side receives reflexive benefits as well.

If you want to massage the other side of her body you have two options: You may reverse her position so that she is lying on her right side facing away from you, repeating the same actions on her opposite side; or you can move to an anterior hold. If you are massaging someone other than your romantic partner or spouse, you will probably find that repeating the posterior hold movements on the opposite side is more comfortable for the receiver.

Benefits of Tantsu

- Enhanced connection
- Increased flexibility
- Relaxation and stress relief
- Intensive nurturing and comfort
- Resetting of the nervous system
- Unwinding of chronic holding patterns
- Supportive of the immune system

Tantsu Anterior Hold

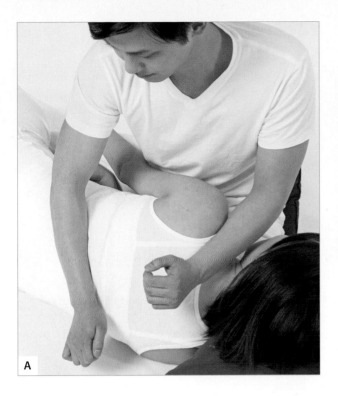

A

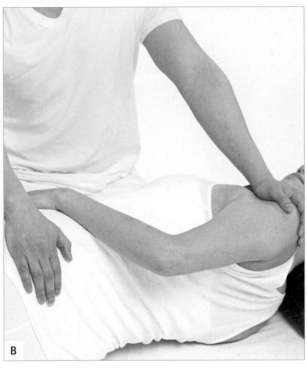

B

Much of what you will do with your partner facing you repeats what you did in the posterior hold but on the other side of her body. One way to release your partner into the anterior position is from a supine position. Place your right thigh between your partner's thighs and roll her toward you or ask her to roll so that her head is once again resting on your left thigh. The second way is to have her sit up, with her right side in front of your chest and her left knee bent and held between her hands, with her left foot on the mat. Support her back and neck as you simultaneously rotate her to face you and lay her head down to your left knee. She will probably have to adjust her position to be fully comfortable with either transition. Use a cushion between her knees and anywhere else it will contribute to her comfort and one or two under your left knee. Cradle her with your left forearm around her shoulder and your right forearm at her hip.

1. ROLL THE SHOULDER, HIP, AND BACK

Allow your partner's breath to move your arms in and out. When your forearms seem to be invited to move, explore her upper shoulder and hip areas with rolling movements (photo A). Gradually work into her lower and middle back with your right forearm. Arriving at her upper back, press against her upper chest next to the deltoid with your left forearm while pulling toward you with your right forearm (photo B). Explore movement by rotating her shoulder as it is contained between your forearms. Her arm may drop behind her so you may want to add a pillow under her elbow. Using your right thumb along points on the medial border of her shoulder blade, press or roll it onto your thumb by rocking the shoulder back with your left forearm or hand. Continuing to press away from you with your left hand on her shoulder, use your right hand to pull her lower back toward you. Hold the twist for a few breaths.

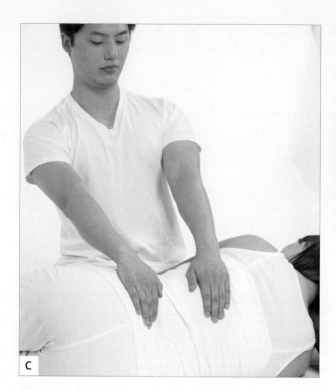

C

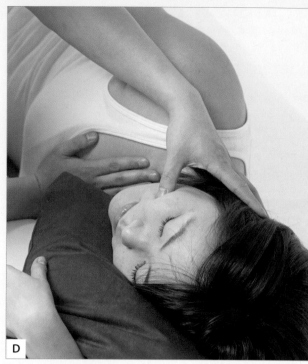

D

2. ROCK THE BACK AND CONNECT THE HEART

Allow your left hand to join your right hand on your partner's back, with your fingers near her spine, and pull toward you, starting near the scapulas and gradually moving down to her low back (**photo C**); with each exhalation you lean back and pull, and on the inhalations you rock forward. You may explore moving up and down her back with your hands moving close together and farther apart. When your right hand reaches her sacrum press into the indentations; then hold your hand over the sacrum and place your left hand on your partner's heart. Hold for several breaths, connecting the heart center with the lower body.

3. CONNECT THE HEAD, STRETCH THE NECK

Keeping your left hand on your partner's heart, with each exhalation press points on her face (detailed in chapter 8), starting with the point at the bridge of the nose; then press under her cheekbone and end with the point just lateral to her eyebrow. Place your right hand on her cheek, in two or three positions, moving your hand toward the back of her head and holding each time for a breath or two (**photo D**).

Massage and Compress the Neck and Shoulder

When the heel of your right hand is on your partner's occiput, move your left hand from her heart to her neck and while you support her head at the occiput with your right hand, move your left hand down her neck, exploring and kneading her neck muscles as you go. When your right hand reaches her shoulder, press it down toward her waist, to give the lateral neck a good stretch, holding for a few breaths (**photo E**). You may knead or just compress her upper shoulder after the stretch, noticing where tension is held and allowing it a few minutes to melt by compressing or squeezing her shoulder, upper arm, and neck (**photo F, page 168**).

Shoulder Tension Reflief

Most people carry a lot of tension in the upper shoulders from driving, carrying, lifting, and working at keyboards that are so high they have to elevate their shoulders. Use both hands to wring the shoulder and open the chest to release this tension.

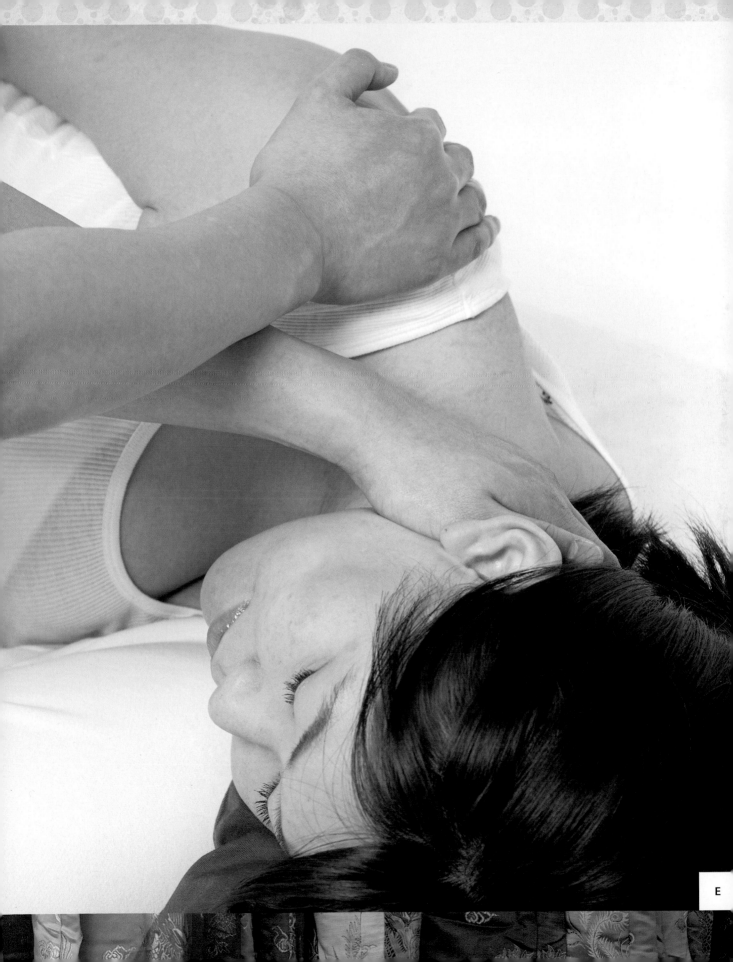

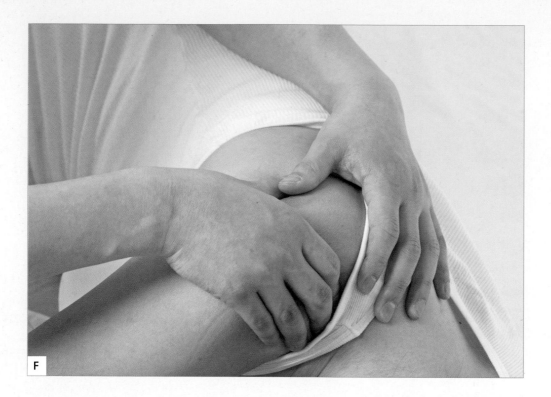

F

4. MASSAGE THE ARM, WRIST, AND HAND

Place your partner's arm on her side while beginning to work down the arm. Squeeze her arm with each exhalation as you move down toward her hand, as though you are squeezing the breath out of her arm (photo G). Lift the weight of her arm in your hands and begin to explore movement with it. You may place your left hand behind her shoulder and take her wrist in your right hand to rotate the shoulder and wrist joints, encouraging increased range of motion and easing tension and strain from heavy work and recreational activities. Place the back of her wrist on her waist and carefully explore how much movement is available in the elbow. Rotate her wrist and work the palm and back of her hand, providing relief to the many small muscles that create the fine dexterity of the hand and which become fatigued from repetitive small movements such as working at a keyboard, playing musical instruments, or writing.

Squeeze and Cradle the Upper Arm

Stretch your partner's arm overhead, placing the back of her hand on the mat, and squeeze the posterior arm muscles, or triceps, with each exhalation. Leaving her arm overhead, cross your arms and stretch the side of her body, holding for a few breaths. Cradle her extended arm, resting on your shoulder, and work the front of the shoulders, upper arm muscles, and chest. If you rotate your torso while cradling her arm, it will stretch the whole shoulder girdle.

Making a Palm-to-Palm Connection

When you release your partner's arm from the cradling, place it on your lower leg and stretch her palm and fingers, rotating her wrist; then place her palm on your heart and your palm on her. Place her palm over your own palm on her heart center and bring your right hand to her hara. Hold for several breaths in stillness. This is a very connecting hold.

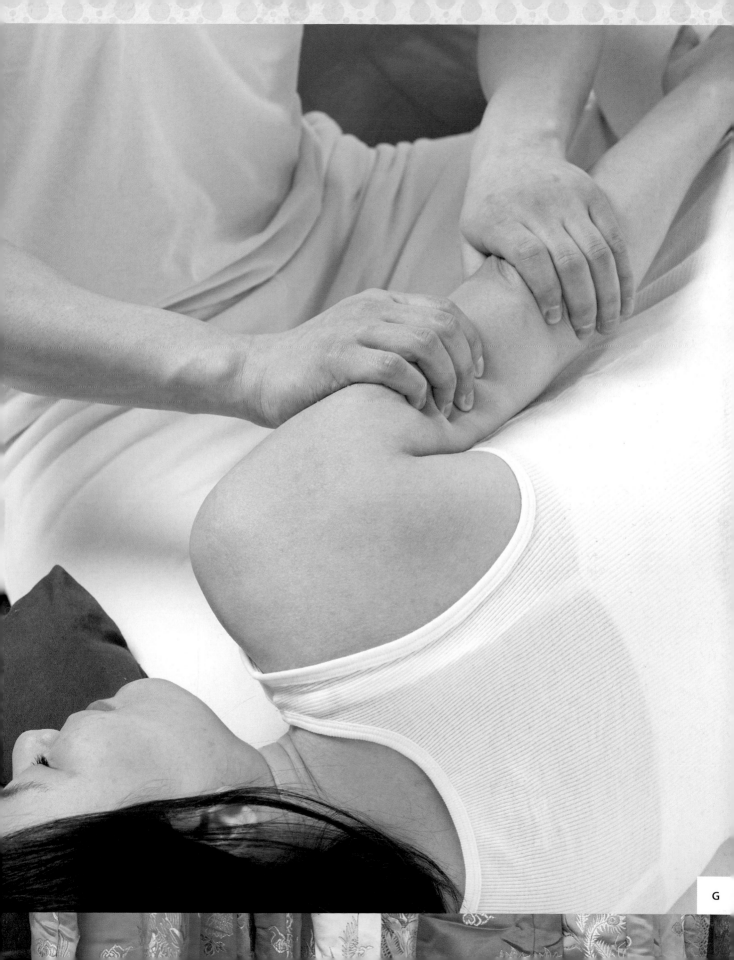

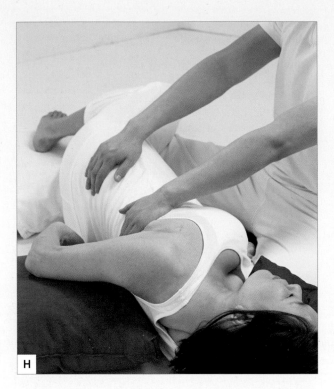

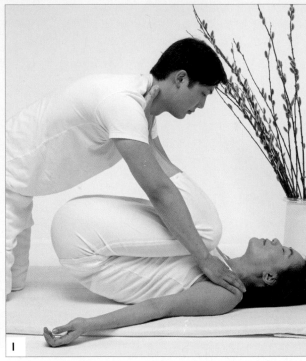

5. LENGTHEN THE BACK, LEG, AND HIP

In the anterior hold, you have the option of allowing your partner's left arm to rest on a cushion behind her back while you rock her toward you with both hands together just above the spine, then with your hands moving farther apart, as your right hand travels down to her hip (photo H). You may use your forearms and hands to roll her hip and thigh areas as you did in the posterior hold and your hands to press in the hollows around her sacrum. If your relative sizes allow you to reach her foot, you may use it to flex her knee toward your left shoulder, allowing you access to her foot and lower leg to knead, wring, and compress as you did on her other side.

6. FINISH WITH STRETCHING AND COMPRESSION

Roll your partner into a supine position, moving all cushions out of the way. Kneel at her feet and bring both of her knees toward her chest, gently leaning your weight on them with your chest on her feet and your hands on her shoulders (photo I). When you extend her legs, squat and lean away from her, creating length as you stretch her legs. Placing her feet back onto the mat, press the arches with your palms and hold; then move up to her hips and press on each hip with your palms, opening the hip joint outward (photo J). Place a hand on her hara for a few breaths. Take her arms over her head and stretch them by leaning your body weight away from her.

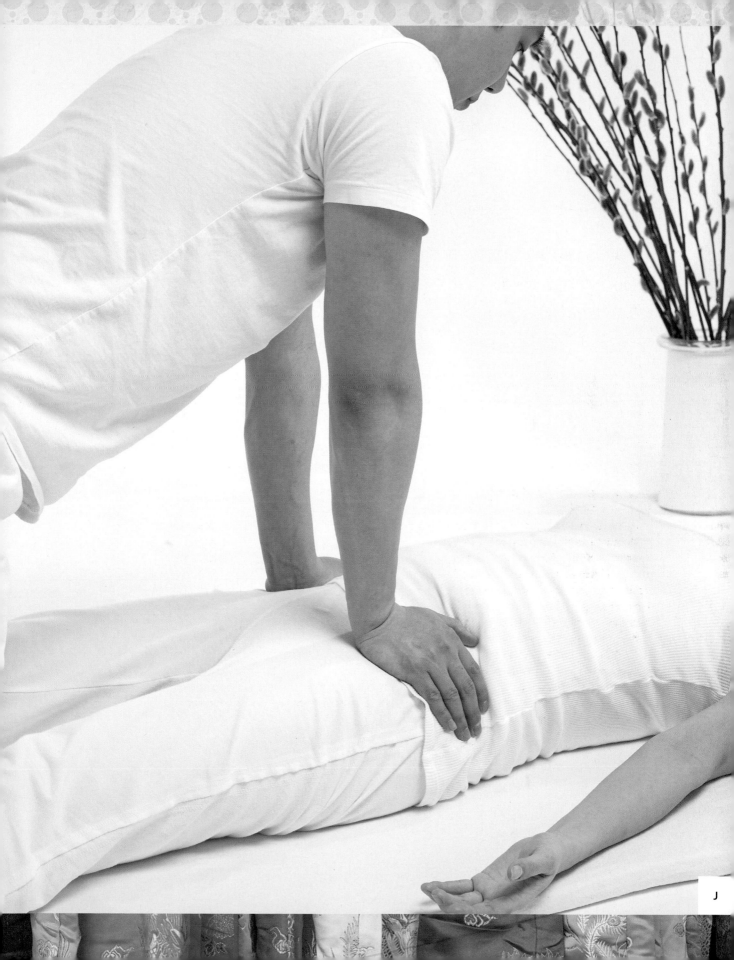

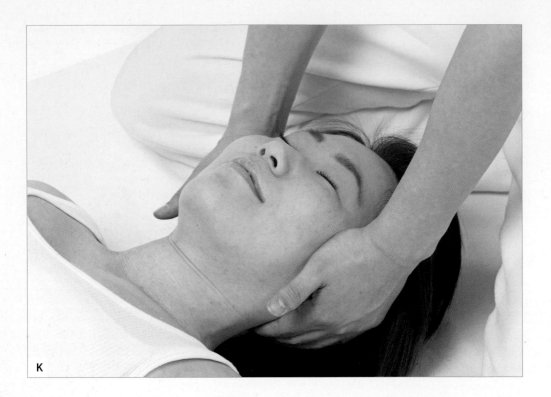

K

7. REST YOUR HANDS ON THE FACE AND HEART

Take a seat at your partner's head and hold at her occipital ridge with your fingers, leaning back to stretch her neck, holding for a few breaths or until she sighs (photo K). This relieves compression and any remaining tension in the neck. Cup your hands over her eyes, but with no pressure on the eyes, covering most of her face with your hands and shutting out light. Take a few breaths. Place your left hand on her forehead and your right hand on her heart with your fingers pointing toward her feet, connecting her head and heart centers for several breaths (photo L). Allow your hands to float up at the end of one of her inhalations and to rest in a seated posture at her head. Feel the connection that remains between you even though you are no longer touching and allow her time to surface from the session.

Learn More about Tantsu

The positions presented here as well as Tantsu's additional positions and moves are included in Harold Dull's book, Tantsu® A Yoga of the Heart, and her DVDs. You can find these, as well as information on Tantsu classes, at www.tantsu.com.

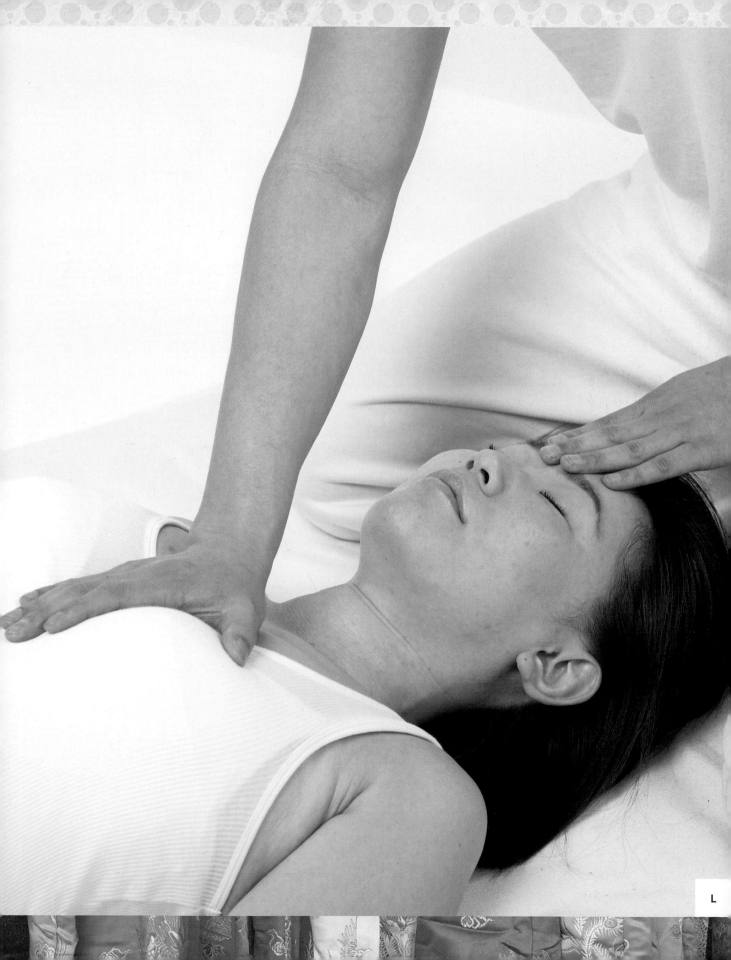

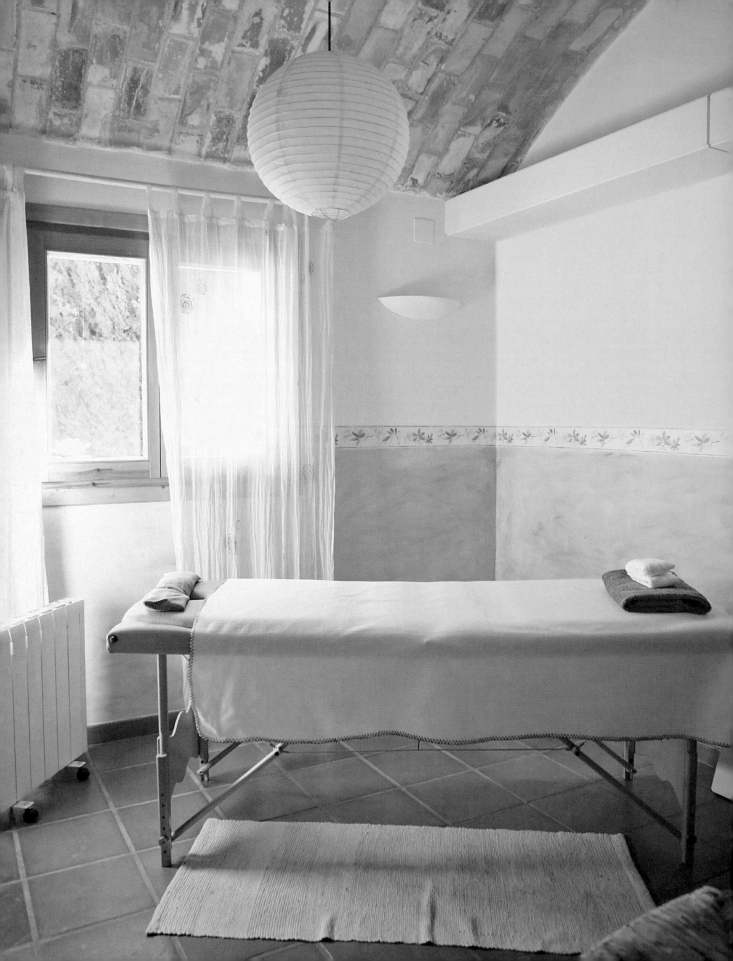

CHAPTER 7

Polarity Clears Physical and Emotional Blocks

Polarity therapy is an integrated, holistic, and hands-on approach to restoring balance to the mind and body through complementary therapeutic methods. One principle of polarity is that the body has poles—hence the name. There is a positive charge toward the top of the body (superior) and a negative charge toward the feet (inferior). The right side is positive and the left is negative. The instructions for polarity sessions are based on using your right hand on the left side of your partner's body and vice versa or your left hand (negative) on his head (positive) and your right hand at his feet.

Rub Hands and Radiate

To get a sense for the feeling of energy, rub your hands together vigorously. Then hold your hands about 6 inches (15.2 cm) apart, preferably with your eyes closed to facilitate your focus on the sensations in your hands. Slowly bring your palms toward each other and feel changes as they come nearer. Sensations may feel like "dense" air between the palms, increased tingling, warmth, or a drawing together of the palms. Moving your hands closer and then farther apart will help you to explore sensations of energy. Explore taking your palms out of direct alignment with each other, then bringing them back, feeling the connection as a "plugged-in" feeling.

Another way to train your awareness of energy is to perform this exercise with your partner or another person and then discuss the sensations each of you felt as your palms moved closer together and farther apart. You may add another dimension as one of you alternately focuses attention fully on the partner's energy, then withdraws focus by taking the mind away—thinking, planning, or remembering something unrelated, then returning to focused attention. Usually the receiver in this exercise will feel the withdrawal of focused attention.

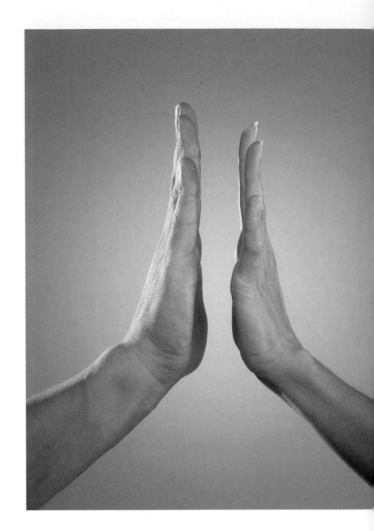

The Vital Principles of Polarity

- The only disease is life-energy disturbance.
- All life is an expression of energy in motion; the body is a system of energies which, when flowing freely, can sustain and nurture itself.
- Optimal health recognizes the interconnectedness of all aspects of life.
- Quality health care is a result of a mind, body, and spirit approach.
- Rocking stimulates life energy.

Preparation for Polarity

Polarity is usually practiced on a person who is dressed but barefoot and wearing no metal jewelry. It may be done with your partner seated in a chair or lying on a massage table or a floor mat. Kneeling on the mat for the relatively short period of time required to perform a polarity session shouldn't be too difficult on your knees, but if you have limited flexibility, use a pillow between your thighs and your calves. You may sit in a cross-legged position when you are working on your partner's head, neck, and face.

The receiver frequently attains a light, trance-like state, an important antidote to routine stress and its wear and tear on the body, mind, and emotions. It may be useful to notice particular holding patterns of muscular tension, movements that suggest stiffness in joints, or other unique characteristics your partner is displaying before you give his a polarity session. Your observations may help you decide where his body may welcome additional energetic input.

Polarity Pressure and Movements

- Pressure, unless otherwise noted, is gentle and light, just the weight of your hands.
- Before each movement, rub your hands together vigorously to charge them with energy. After each movement, throw static energy off by flicking your hands as though you are flicking water.
- Remain in each position for one or two minutes or until you feel your partner's relaxation reaching a plateau rather than continuing to deepen.
- Rocking movements start small and build into larger rocking. When rocking, press away and let your partner's body come back at its own rate, setting the rhythm. Rock from your feet, transmitting the movement from your whole body, not just your arms.
- Remain alert and focused on what you feel and sense in your partner's body. Have no agenda for "fixing" anything; be an accepting witness for the body.
- Remain relaxed and comfortable in your own body and stance or you may transmit tension into your partner's body.
- Invite and encourage relaxation; don't be disappointed if some areas resist relaxation.

The Polarity Sequence

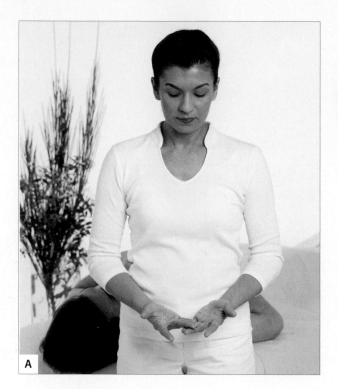

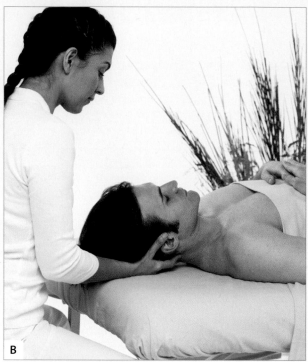

You don't have to follow this general sequence, but it is thought to be more effective if you follow the order given. Polarity sessions always start and end at the head. A polarity session usually lasts between thirty and forty-five minutes.

1. CRADLE THE HEAD, STRETCH THE NECK

Have your partner lie face up (supine) on a massage table. Sit on a stool or chair at the head of the table at a height that allows your shoulders to relax with your forearms resting on the table. Overlap the lateral three fingers of your left hand over the same fingers of your right hand to form a cradle (**photo A**). Your index fingers will rest in the hollow right below the lateral occipital ridge at the base of your partner's skull, just behind his ears (**photo B**). Hold this position for about two minutes, as your partner's breathing slows and deepens.

Keep your right hand under his neck, palm up, and put your left hand on his forehead. Exert a gradual, steady pull on his neck, inviting length. Do not lift his head but keep your hand on the surface of the table (**photo C**). This stretch creates a welcome feeling of openness in the neck and helps release tight neck muscles that can result in headaches and neck pain.

2. ROCK THE BELLY

Stand at your partner's left side. Bring your right hand slowly down and place your palm on his abdomen, below his navel. Sense any tension and changes in breathing patterns throughout the session. The body seems to have its own sensibility, and when an area feels "heard" frequently, it will relax and reorganize into a more healthful configuration. The abdomen is an especially energy-sensitive part of the body, so listen carefully with your hands to its responses.

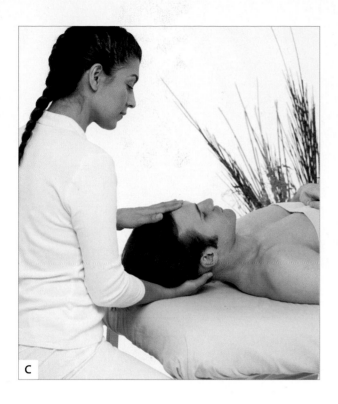

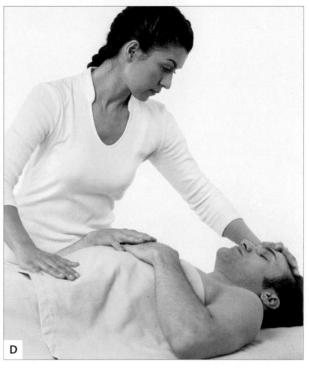

With your right hand still on his abdomen, place your left hand gently on his forehead (**photo D**). Notice whether you feel the connection of energy in your hands. Begin to rock his lower body, like rocking an infant, and gradually make the movements larger. His body will return on its own and establish the rhythm; allow it to lead the dance. Continue rocking for a few minutes, feeling tension seep out of his body, possibly noticing a freer flow of energy, increased color in his face, and deeper breathing.

You will notice a sinking into a plateau of relaxation each time there is completion in any area. Releasing tension in the abdomen can reduce symptoms of irritable bowel syndrome, Crohn's disease, indigestion, nausea, constipation, and acid reflux. Emotions such as fear are often held in the belly and may be relieved through the kind of relaxation and energetic balancing that polarity provides.

Warning! Nonattachment Required

The mindset for giving a polarity session is relaxed and loving. You should not attempt to give a polarity session if you have negative feelings toward your receiver or if you are ill, tired, spaced out, or emotionally upset. We tend to be less than optimal conduits for life energy when we are not feeling well. It is possible to "pick up" less than optimal energy from another person, although generally, energy is neutral. Some people feel they have uncomfortable bodily or emotional feelings following a session on a receiver who is ill, demanding, or expressing negativity in some way. Generally, you will not acquire negative feelings or symptoms if you are not attached to fixing or healing the person who is receiving polarity.

Lift the Hip to Open the Pelvis

Notice whether your partner's feet are turned laterally (toes facing outward), and if they are, reach under his body, with one hand well under his waist and the other under his hip. Lift and pull his hip outward and then move your hand positions to his hip and upper thigh and repeat the outward pull (**photo E**). This will create a feeling of space in the hips and pelvis and will roll the leg into a more neutral position, with the foot facing upward. Move to the right side of his body and repeat.

This move reminds the body that openness can exist in the posterior pelvis and releases unconscious holding patterns. A person may hold strong emotions in this area from having been spanked as a child or from having fallen on his backside repeatedly. Polarity can infuse balanced energy to help dissipate some of the fearful feelings and holding in the buttocks.

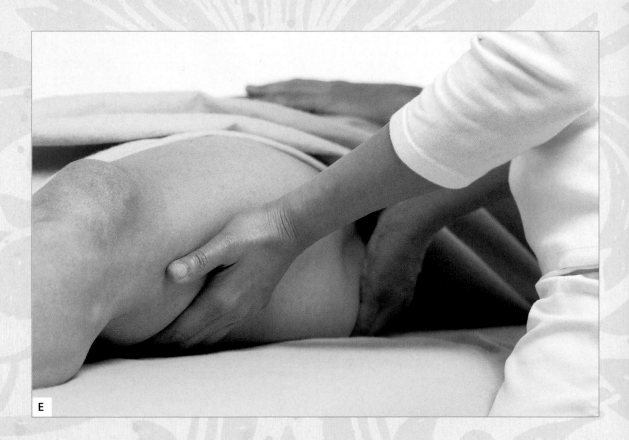

E

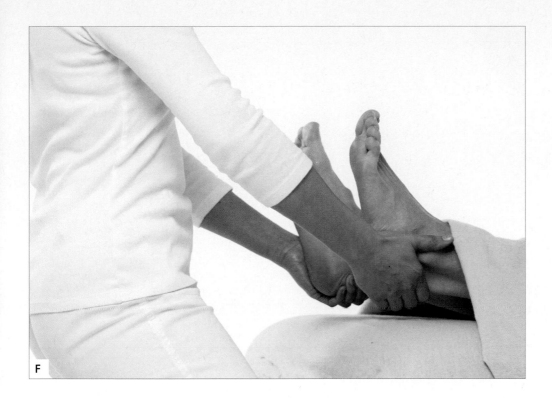

F

3. PULL THE LEGS TO OPEN CHANNELS OF ENERGY

Come to the foot of the table, bringing your stool or chair. Starting at your partner's right thigh, sweep your hands all the way down his leg and off the toes a few times, shaking your hands off at the end of each sweep, and then repeat with his other leg. This is an energy sweep that prepares the legs for deeper work and loosens the strong weight-bearing joints of the lower limb.

Take his heels in your hands. Hold the wide part of his heels, not compressing the narrow Achilles tendon above the heel. Lean back slowly, putting some tension on his legs and lifting them slightly above the level of the table as you lean back (**photo F**). Again, this move comes from your whole body, all the way down to your feet, rather than just the arms; it decompresses the hip and knee joints. Opening the channels of energy that flow through the knees may assist in decompressing that joint and reduce symptoms of locking, crepitus (popping), stiffness, and discomfort.

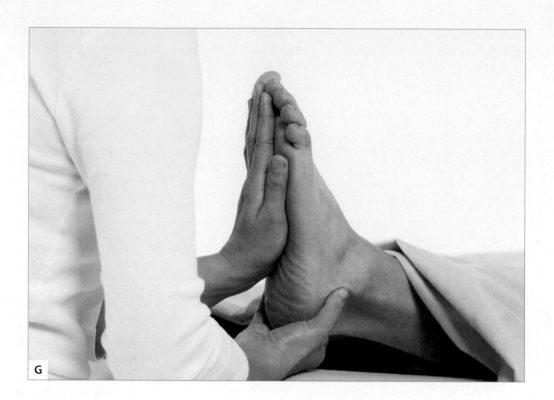

G

4. WAKE UP THE FEET, LEGS, AND PELVIS

Sit on the stool and wake up your partner's feet by vigorously rocking his right forefoot, then his left, between loose hands. Place the palm of your right hand under his right heel and the palm of your left hand on the ball of his foot. Lean forward, dorsiflexing his foot, bringing the top of his foot toward his shin (photo G). Press the top of his foot downward toward the table (plantarflexion), leaning back to create some traction. Rotate his foot with your left hand, still holding his heel in your right hand. These movements of the ankles will increase flexibility and allow a freer flow of energy through the joint. Dorsiflex his foot again, using your right thumb to press in a circle from slightly in front of the medial malleolis, or ankle bone, to below and behind it, pressing all around the medial heel with each dorsiflexion of the foot.

Switch hands, pressing against the ball of his foot with your right hand. With your left hand under his heel, perform compressions and circles around the outside or lateral malleolis and heel with your left thumb. These moves address heel discomfort and have reflexive effects in the lower body (see chapter 5); they are particularly useful for alleviating menstrual cramps in women.

Gently Pull the Toes

Hold the front of your partner's foot with your left hand and gently pull each toe, starting with the big toe. This is a sustained, slow pull. It may release trapped energy in the joints, causing some toes to crack, but that is not the purpose of the pulls, so be gentle. Each toe has its own energy charge.

Repeat all of the foot actions on your partner's left foot. After completing his left foot, place your fingertips on the tips of all ten toes and feel for an even sensation of energy from each toe. If any toe feels less "awake" than others, you may return to that area and repeat the toe pulls. Hold both feet lightly for a few moments

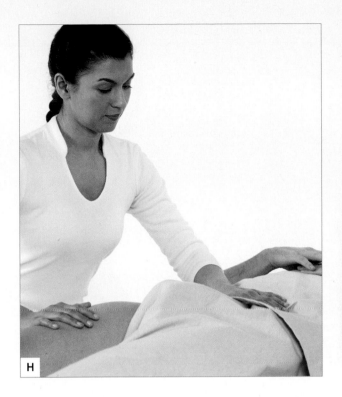

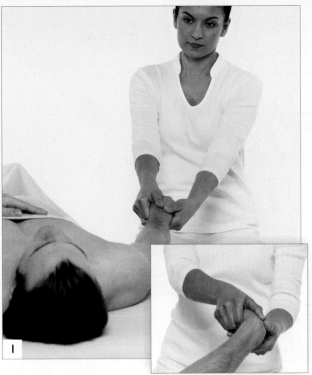

to end the section. You have encouraged life energy to flow upward from the feet and have made energy available for these hard-working parts of the body. Adequate energy in the feet can contribute to stronger arches, thus helping alleviate arch and foot pain that can translate all the way up through the legs and into the hips and back.

Rock the Leg and Pelvis

Standing at your partner's right hip, place your right hand just above his knee and your left hand on his lower abdomen. Slowly begin to rock his left leg, pushing it away using your whole body and then allowing it to rebound at its own rate **(photo H)**. Rock his leg in a flowing rhythm for up to a minute; then maintain stillness with your hands in the same positions. Notice the quality of energy you feel before and after the rocking.

5. ARM, HAND, FINGER, AND SHOULDER MOVEMENTS

Hold your partner's wrist between your thumbs and fingers, with your thumbs on top of his wrist. While leaning back, put some gentle traction on his arm, with his elbow lifted above the table surface **(photo I)**. Take his flexed wrist toward his shoulder and bring it back toward you in a flowing movement. Continue with the fluid movement, also adding medial and lateral movement into the circular motion **(photo insert)**, for about a minute. These motions will enhance flexibility in the wrist, elbow, and shoulder joints. Regular polarity sessions integrating these hand, arm, and shoulder movements may assist in preventing some repetitive strain injuries from occurring due to overuse in work or hobbies.

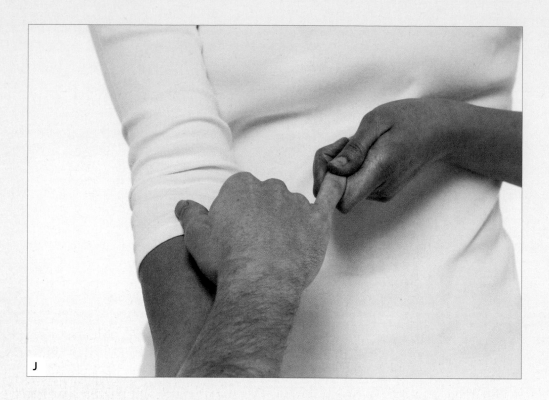

J

Pull Fingers and Pause

After holding your partner's hand in the same position for a few moments, grasp the web between his thumb and forefinger between your right thumb and forefinger and place your left hand 1 inch (2.5 cm) below his elbow crease, toward the lateral side of his arm. Alternate pressure on the two points for about a minute, keeping soft thumbs; then hold in stillness. Still holding his elbow, give each finger and his thumb a gradual pull, with his forearm off the table surface, releasing tension held in his hands and fingers (**photo J**). Facing your partner's head, lightly grasp his right elbow with your palm facing upward and your thumb slightly above the elbow crease. Place your right hand along his left lower rib cage.

6. ROCK THE TORSO

Begin to alternate strokes: a small upward stroke with your thumb, rocking your partner's torso away from you (**photo K**). Put your right hand on his upper abdomen and your thumb just below his lateral clavicle. Use both hands to establish rocking of his torso, moving your thumb medially and laterally as you do so. This move may open the chest and give the receiver a sense of more openness and room to breathe in the chest.

Place your left hand on his right hip and rock his left shoulder with your right hand. Continue this rhythm for about a minute; then continue the hold in stillness for another minute.

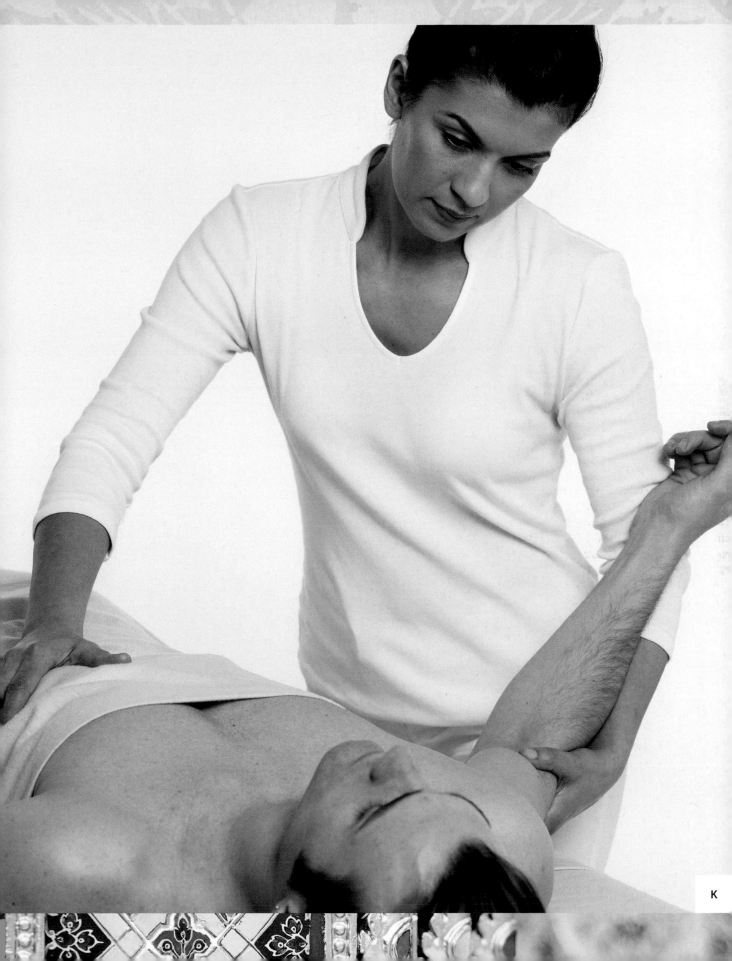

Sense Energy and Breath

Hold your partner's right hand in your left hand and his left foot in your right hand. No movement is required; just sense his energy and notice his breath. Move to the opposite side of the table and repeat the sequence from the leg and pelvis rock through the hand/foot hold.

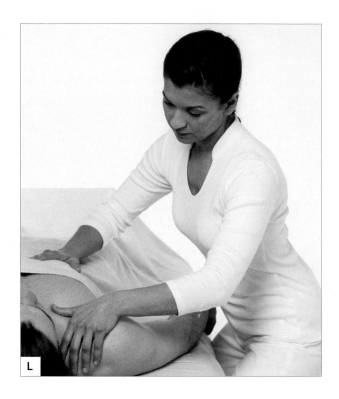

L

Benefits of Polarity

- Promotes a feeling of being filled with energy
- Relaxes muscle tension
- Stimulates the parasympathetic nervous system for renewal and repair
- Slows the heart rate
- Slows and deepens respiration
- Lowers blood pressure
- Reduces pain
- Improves circulation
- Increases endorphin production
- Promotes healing through balanced energy
- Improves digestion
- Normalizes hormone levels

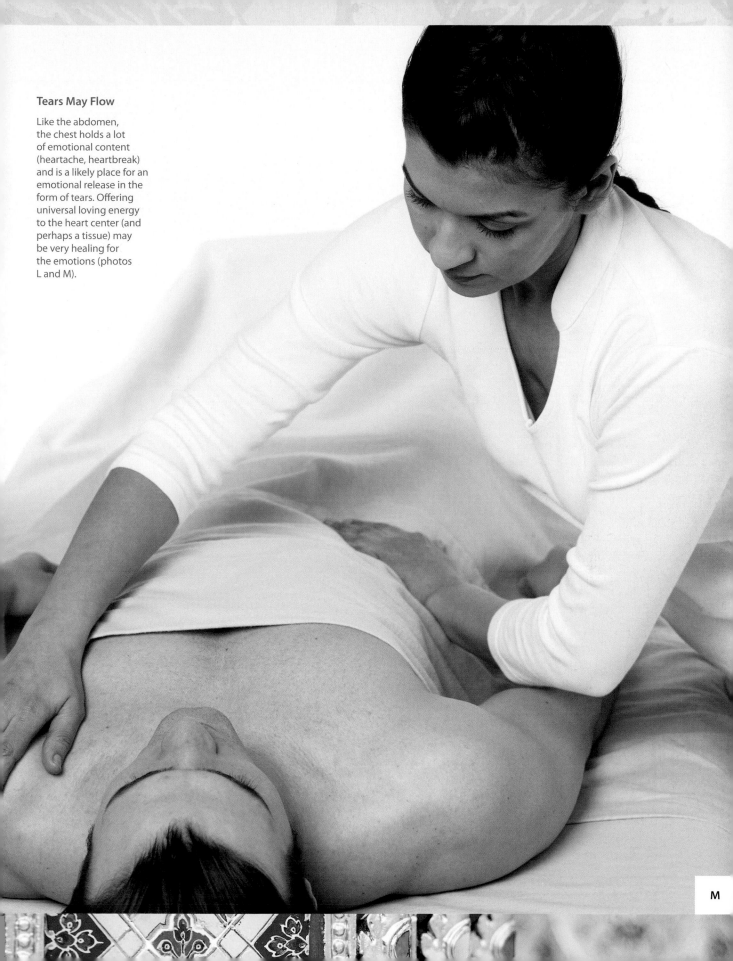

Tears May Flow

Like the abdomen, the chest holds a lot of emotional content (heartache, heartbreak) and is a likely place for an emotional release in the form of tears. Offering universal loving energy to the heart center (and perhaps a tissue) may be very healing for the emotions (photos L and M).

M

7. HOLD THE HEAD, NECK, AND FACE

Sitting at the head of the table, tilt your partner's head about forty-five degrees to the right, with your right hand resting softly on his forehead (**photo N**). With your left middle finger supported by your other fingers, press the lateral occipital ridge (where you held on each side for the head cradle). Hold the position for close to two minutes and repeat on the opposite side. This position puts a nice stretch on the lateral neck and calms energy in the head, often reducing headache discomfort. The stretch can improve space for the brachia plexus, a bundle of nerves and blood vessels that serves the whole arm and hand, reducing symptoms of numbness, tingling, weakness, and pain deep in the forearm.

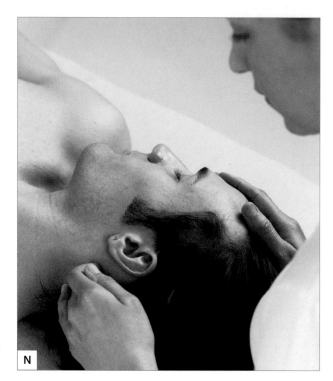

N

With your partner's head and neck in a neutral position again, place both of your index fingers on the middle forehead slightly above the level of his eyebrows (the third eye) and your other three fingertips spread along his forehead. While your fingers are pressing the facial points, your thumbs are pressing directly downward at the top of his head (the anterior fontanel). Hold for about two minutes, noticing any unevenness in the pulsations for energy from one side of his head and face to the other. This position can calm the spirit and may relieve headaches, both tension and sinus in origin. If your partner is suffering from sinus congestion, you may want to hold points below his cheekbone, right below his pupils.

OPTIONAL SPINAL HOLD

You may add a spinal hold at this point in the sequence. Ask your partner to turn over, with his head in a face cradle. From his left side, place your right hand on his sacrum and your left hand on his upper back (**photo O**). Rock his sacrum away from you for about two minutes, allowing his rhythm to inform the movement. This optional movement is useful for reducing back pain by increasing flexibility and movement in the spine and pelvic girdle and can stimulate stronger energy in the vertebral column, supporting upright posture.

Return to your partner's right side and place your left hand on his forehead and your right hand over his heart, but not touching his body. Remember the strong emotional content in this area and endeavor to connect to that with your loving energy. Hold this position for at least two minutes; then slowly remove your hands and let your partner rest for a few minutes. When he is ready to sit up, have him sit on the edge of the table, with his feet supported in a chair.

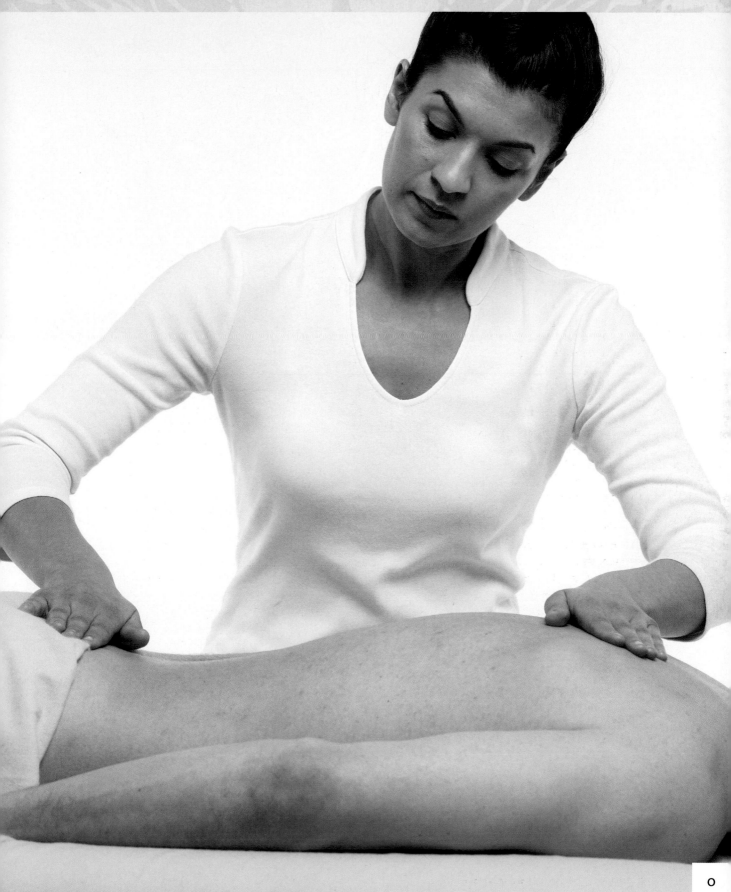

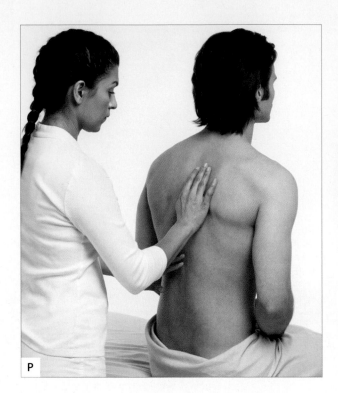

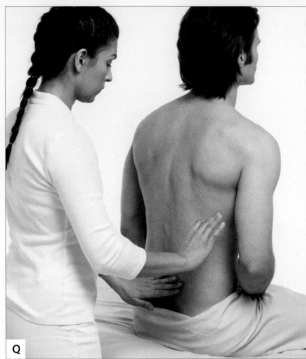

CLOSING SWEEPS

Stand with your hands on your partner's shoulders and sweep your hands medially, crossing one hand over the other between his shoulder blades **(photo P)** and continuing the sweep down his back **(photo Q)**. When your hands reach his waist, your hands will sweep out to his hips with your arms no longer crossed **(photo R)**. Shake the energy off at the end of each sweep and perform about ten repetitions; then move out to his hips. Each sweep should be lighter in pressure than the preceding one.

Come to a standing position in front of your partner and be sure his hands are resting on his thighs. Sweep from the top of his head, down his neck and shoulders, and all the way out to his fingertips. Sweep from the top of his head down his legs to his feet. Repeat these steps, alternating between sweeping the arms and the legs, about ten times. Sweeping clears the energy field of static and feels very nurturing to the receiver. There should be no agenda about the end result of a polarity session. Just relax and be open, placing your hands on your partner in a giving way. In polarity, we are passively channeling and concentrating the energy of the universe through our bodies while intuitively sensing where there are blockages, shortages, or excess energy. There is no need for strain or effort; your partner will draw into himself what his body needs to balance his energy. You can trust the body's intelligence to use energy wisely, so perform the work with loving ease and comfort.

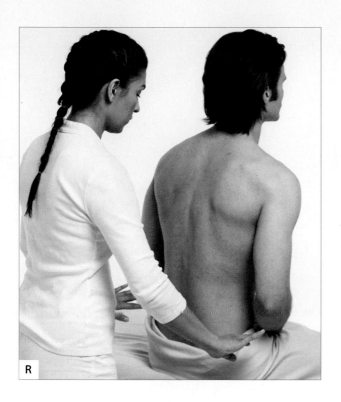

R

A Glass of Water Would Be Nice

You will want to offer your partner water after the polarity session and be sure he is grounded before driving or operating equipment. It will be optimal if he can simply relax after receiving a session.

Use Polarity with Swedish Massage

It is easy to integrate polarity into a Swedish massage on the table, and many massage therapists routinely include some polarity in their bodywork sequences. You may choose to integrate a particular polarity hold or rocking action when you perceive from massage that an area of energy is blocked or has an overabundance of intense energy. Polarity is particularly easy on the hands and can offer a break from the stronger exertions characteristic of various forms of massage.

Emotional and Spiritual Concerns

The kind of energy healing polarity offers does not differentiate between mind and body. Some people may experience spaciousness and a connection to you or to the universe or a higher power. Enjoy basking in their wonder and sharing the special time and avoid taking any credit for the energy for which you have been a conduit. Often, those receiving a polarity session will have issues from the past or the present bubble to the surface of their consciousness during a session. If this happens, allow them to talk about their feelings. Be open and accepting and if possible, reflect directly back to them what they say to you, as they may be in a trance-like condition and it may help them to keep their thoughts organized to hear them repeated back. When they have finished what they have to say you can move on to the next hand position in the sequence. They may or may not choose to share what their experiences were, emotionally or spiritually, during a session, and this must be honored.

AN INSIDE JOB

Healing comes from within. In polarity, the giver and receiver work together to allow the receiver's inner healing to emerge.

The more you give polarity sessions, the more sensitive you will become to life energy and its movements in others' bodies. The receiver may experience emotions spontaneously or feel the need to talk about his life when tense tissues begin to relax and unwind. You can facilitate this unwinding process by reflecting back your partner's thoughts and emotions as you continue the session. Verbal communication should be nondirective with the intention of helping your partner become aware of his process. At any time, your partner may stop talking and the session will move naturally back into silent bodywork.

For the most part, though, your partner will simply feel a sense of enhanced well-being from a polarity session, and you will reap some of the same benefits by being the conduit through which the intention of balancing energy flows.

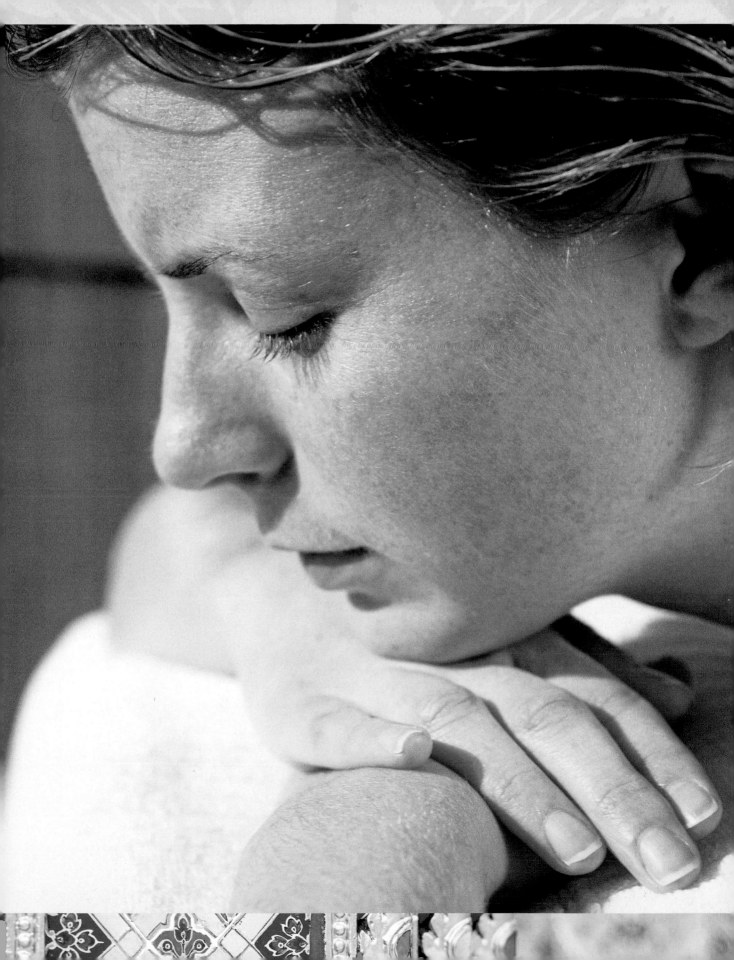

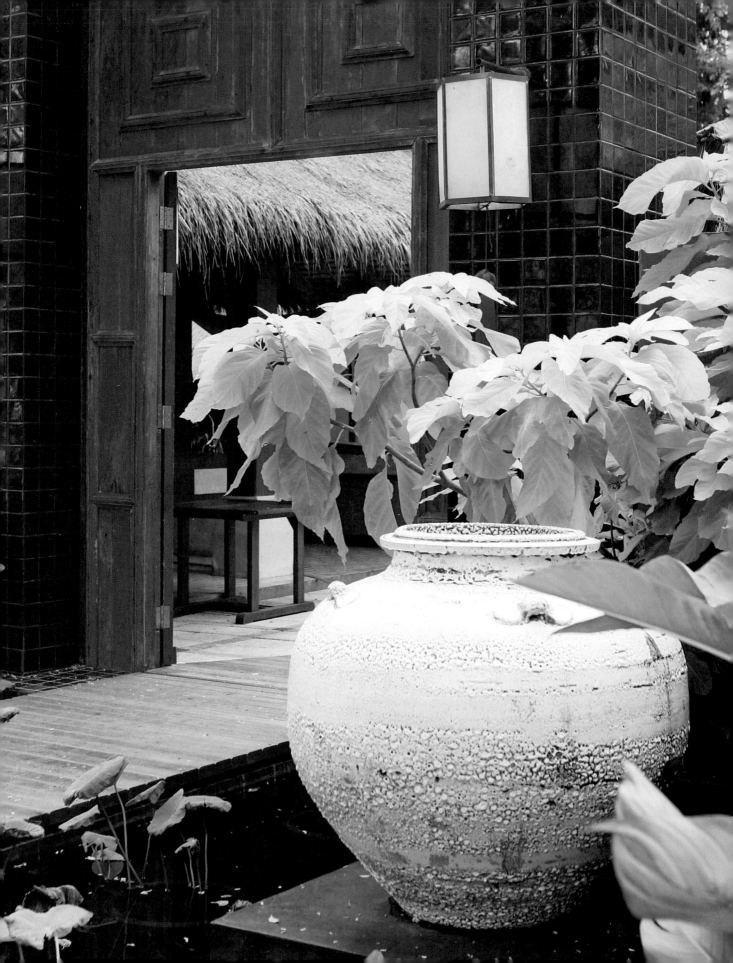

CHAPTER 8

Shiatsu Activates Energy Meridians

Many forms of shiatsu have emerged since 1940, although its roots go back much further in time. In traditional shiatsu, energy lines or meridians that are associated with organs of the body are compressed with fingers and thumbs to promote healing.

Compressing the Meridian Lines

Like acupuncture and acupressure, shiatsu involves stimulation of points along the meridian lines, but the pressure is sometimes applied over a wider area, with palms, forearms, elbows, knees, or feet rather than needles and in addition to precise finger and thumb pressure. Stretching along the meridian lines is also used to address the fourteen meridians in a general way.

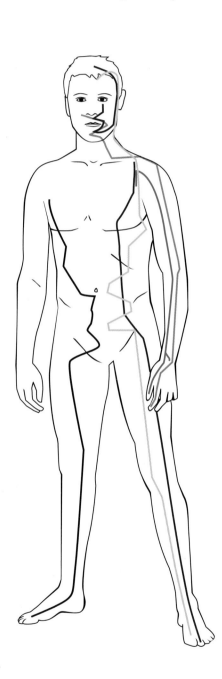

Liver meridian
Digestive problems
Genital/sexual problems
Varicose veins
Gout/ingrown toenails, fungus, etc.

Spleen/pancreas meridian
Abdominal pain
Menstrual pain

Stomach meridian
Lung/bronchial problems
Digestive problems
Thigh/knee pain

Lung meridian
Shoulder pain
Skin problems
Carpal tunnel syndrome

Large intestine (colon) meridian
Bloody nose
Cold sores
Tennis elbow
Arthritis

————— Bladder meridian
Pain and stiffness along spine
Hemorrhoids
Sciatica
Tightness in calf

————— Triple warmer/endocrine/three-E meridian
Shoulder pain
Pain in arm and wrist
Arthritis, warts

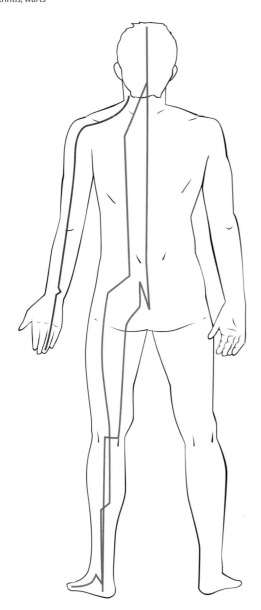

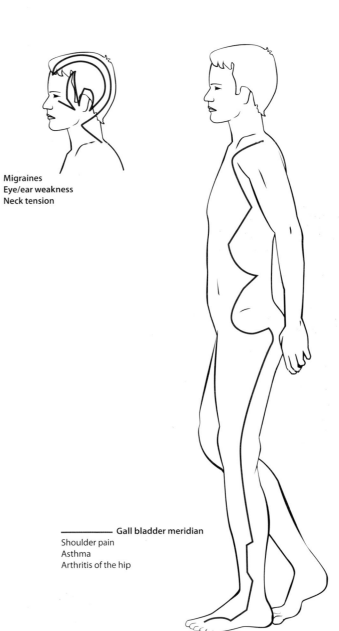

Migraines
Eye/ear weakness
Neck tension

————— Gall bladder meridian
Shoulder pain
Asthma
Arthritis of the hip

QI MOVEMENT: A PRE-SHIATSU EXPLORATION

Relax and position yourself comfortably on your hands and knees, with your knees hip width apart. After finding a really balanced position of ease, move forward and back, consciously playing with the transfer of weight and gradually adding some circular motion. Become very aware of moving from the abdominal center of gravity, or hara, using it to transfer weight from your center into your hands, holding for a few seconds each time the weight is on your hands, coming to the floor, and then onto your partner's body, at right angles. This prepares you to provide optimal compressive qi manipulation.

Next, practice centered movement with one hand on your partner's upper back and the other on his sacrum, rocking your weight forward and holding for a few seconds. Repeat the rocking compressions several times and check with your partner to make sure the pressure is comfortable. Remaining relaxed and using body weight rather than muscular strength is more relaxing for the receiver and less tiring for you.

Preparation for Shiatsu

- Wear comfortable, loose-fitting clothes made of natural fibers, which don't disrupt the flow of energy. Make sure you are centered and grounded before beginning a shiatsu session and that you are ready to fully focus on your partner.
- Provide a firm, padded floor mat measuring at least 4' x 6.5' (1.2 x 2 m) and covered with a clean sheet tucked under so that the surface is smooth. The perimeter should be clear of furniture and other objects for at least 3 feet (91.4 cm) beyond the mat. Have cushions available for bolstering and comfort. The room should be warm, quiet, neat, and clean for optimal energy flow.
- The person receiving shiatsu should not have a large meal before the session.

Shiatsu Pressure and Length of Holds

To thumb points on lines, lean your weight on a thumb or finger, whichever keeps your wrists more neutral, and hold for about three to five seconds or one breath, unless otherwise noted. Apply gentle to moderate pressure with the pad of your thumb or finger rather than the tip. If you are palming an area where your wrist is strongly hyperextended (i.e., toward a right angle with the back of the hand toward the forearm), you may use a loose fist to reduce any strain from applying mild pressure on your wrist.

If thumbing points begins to feel uncomfortable, put your flat thumb on the points and use the pressure from your other hand to create the compression. This may mean you will be unable to thumb two areas at once, but it is far more important to safeguard your hands than to complete a session more quickly. Although a wide range of pressure is applied during professional shiatsu sessions, consider that you are working energetically with meridian lines and that energetic work does not require substantial effort. It is more important to sink in slowly and sensitively than to work deeply.

The spaces between points you are thumbing may be as close together as the distance across your fingertip to 1 inch (2.5 cm) or more apart. In general, use wider spacing to thumb larger areas, such as the legs, compared to the face or neck.

To palm means to apply even pressure with the entire palm on an area. The C hold, used mostly on the limbs, allows for broader stimulation of points and meridian lines on two sides of an arm or leg simultaneously, sinking in as you rock forward with your hand curved so that both your fingers and the heel of your hand are pressing into the muscles. This differs from squeezing pressure, such as petrissage, in that your fingers are curved and the pressure is applied only with fingers and thumbs, rather than with the palms as well.

Shiatsu Sequence

Although the essence of shiatsu combines diagnosis and therapy, you may use an effective basic routine without an in-depth knowledge of the theories and diagnostic techniques if you are willing to focus and develop sensitivity to your partner's energy. A general shiatsu sequence lasting seventy-five minutes or so may enhance wellness and assist recovery from illness by positively stimulating the immune system and natural healing abilities without diagnosing and treating a specific problem. No lubricants or scents are used in shiatsu, and music is employed only if it does not interfere with the coordination of breath and compressions.

1. PRESS POINTS ON THE FACE AND HEAD

With your partner lying supine on the mat, sit or kneel at his head and place your fingers on each side of the head. Use your thumbs to press from the midpoint between his eyebrows toward his hairline (about four to six compressions, about a fingertip distance apart), leaning gently into your thumbs on each exhalation (photo A). Then continue compressions to the crown of his head (the bladder meridian).

Place your index fingers on each side of the bridge of his nose and press toward the bridge (the eye brightener point). Then press with your fingers from the medial eyebrows across his brow to the point where his ear meets his face (photo B). This small indentation at the side of the face in front of the ear is useful for relieving headaches. Using your fingers press from the bridge of his nose along the bone below his eye (bladder meridian) toward his temples.

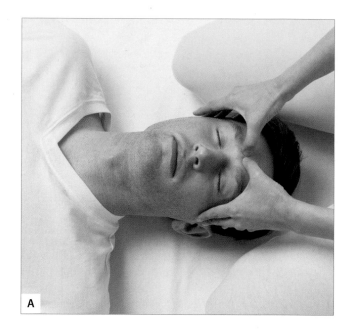

A

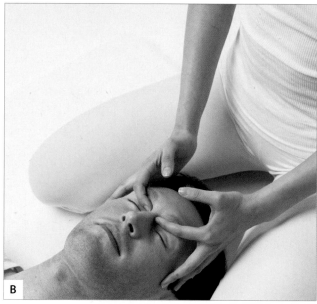

B

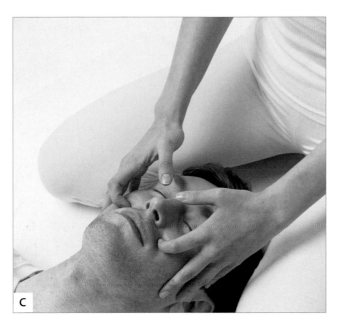

C

Starting with an index finger on either side of his nose crease, press just below his cheekbone on the liver and stomach meridians and out to his ear **(photo C)**. Immediately below his pupil along this line is a stomach point called Facial Beauty which is very useful for relieving sinus pain and congestion. Pause here for a few breaths if that is an issue. End the thumbing at the lateral face indentation in front of his ear (noted earlier) that may relieve headaches with sustained (a few breaths) pressure.

Press one thumb or index finger in the area between your partner's top lip and his nose **(photo D)** on the point called the Middle of a Person on the governing vessel meridian, which is thought to relieve pain, revive consciousness, and reduce fainting and dizziness.

Starting at the center of his chin, pinch along his jaw line laterally to the lateral angle of his jaw. When you arrive at the angle of his jaw, compress or provide friction at the masseter muscle, addressing the Jaw Chariot point on the stomach meridian, which may help with stress, jaw and tooth pain, and TMJ problems.

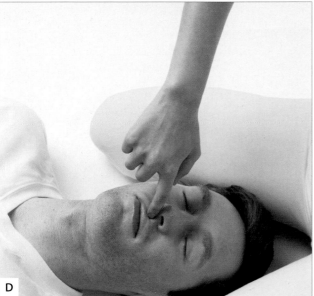

D

Hope for Homeostasis

Treating the body as a whole with shiatsu helps restore the optimal nervous, circulatory, glandular, and metabolic system functions and stimulates homeostasis, a harmony of mind and body. The energetic balancing essence of shiatsu promotes overall balance of mind, body, and spirit, with resultant wellness.

Stretch and Massage the Neck

With one hand on your partner's occiput, stretch his neck to the left and compress his right shoulder at the Shoulder Well, a point on the gallbladder meridian midway between the point of the shoulder and the neck, toward his feet (photo E). Hold for a few breaths and repeat on the other side.

Roll your fingers in a wave-like action up his neck, starting at the base and lifting your fingers against the back of the neck, and then pull them toward you and repeat, gradually working all the way to the occiput. Place your fingers parallel to his spine. Gently lift your partner's head off the mat, tilting his chin slightly toward his chest, which stretches the bladder meridian in the posterior neck. Holding your fingers on the occipital ridge at the base of his skull, lean back and create length in his neck and bladder meridian. Rest the backs of your hands on the mat and make small circles just lateral to his spine, moving up and down his neck from the occipital ridge to his shoulders, following the bladder meridian.

**Warning!
Avoid Palming over
Rigid Contact Lenses**

Be sure you know whether your partner is wearing rigid contact lense and have him remove them or avoid contact in this hold. Place both palms over his eyes, resting gently, with your fingers toward the bridge of his nose. Hold for several breaths. This is very restful for the eyes and is especially important if you notice a lot of eye movement under the lids.

Benefits of Shiatsu

- Provides deep muscle relaxation
- Reduces osteoarthritis pain
- Reduces stress and anxiety
- Releases toxins from the body
- Provides general wellness through energy (qi) balancing
- Increases flexibility
- Improves blood and lymph circulation
- Reduces blood pressure

- Reduces PMS symptoms
- Improves sleep and reduces fatigue
- Reduces muscle and joint pain
- Increases mental and spiritual awareness
- Improves digestion
- Eases depression
- Assists in recovery from injuries
- Provides general well-being and pleasure

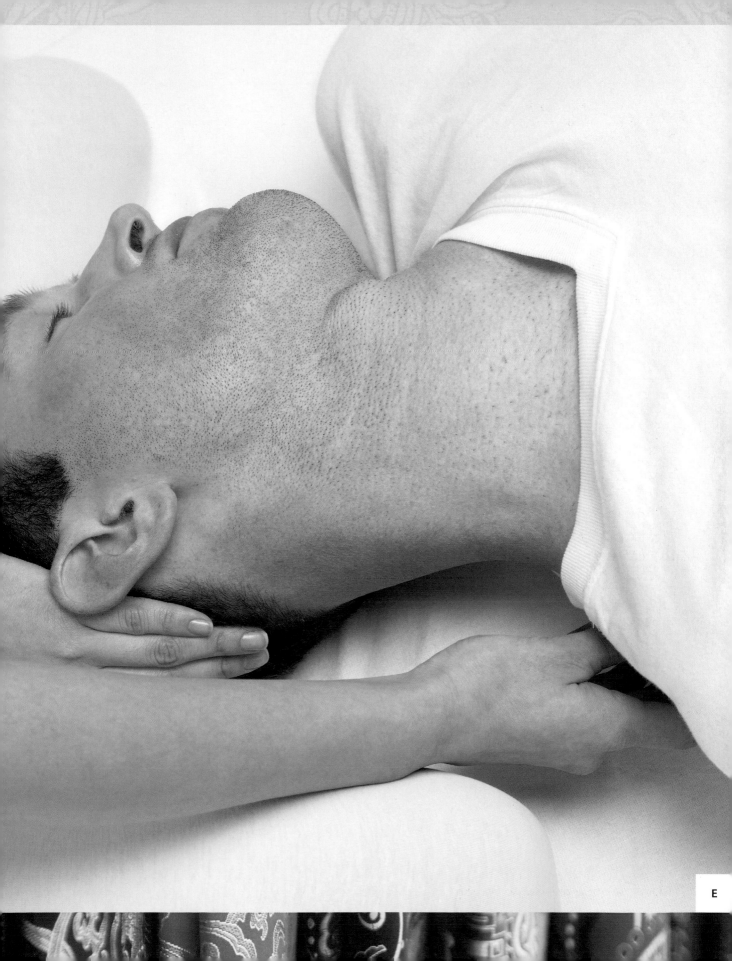

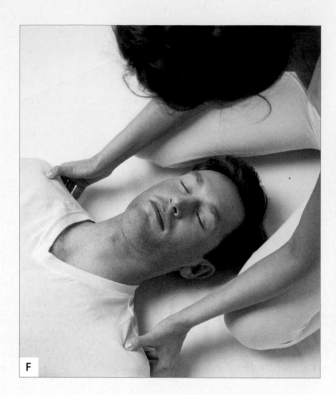

F

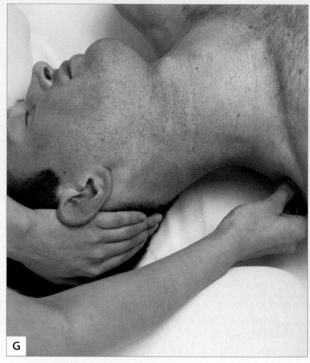

G

2. COMPRESS THE SHOULDERS, CHEST, AND ABDOMEN

Scoop your hands under your partner's shoulders, palms up, and press your arms down on the mat, compressing upward with your fingers between his spine and shoulder blades. Perform circular friction along the medial borders of his shoulder blades (scapulas) to their upper angles.

Thumb deeply, one press per exhalation, from the top of his shoulders next to his neck, out to the flat bone near the lateral point of his shoulder, pausing on the Shoulder Well point, and out to the acromium process, the flat bone at the lateral point of the shoulder (**photo F**).

Return to his neck, which should be softer and more relaxed, making it possible to compress more deeply. Use either finger presses or circular friction to work from his shoulders to the occipital ridge (**photo G**), pausing about 1 inch (2.5 cm) before the ridge on the band of muscle just lateral to the spine; these points reduce irritability, fatigue, and nervousness. Curl your fingers at the base of the occiput and hold for a few breaths. The points on the muscle at the occipital ridge running just laterally to the spine are called the Gates of Consciousness and can relieve neck stiffness and pain, headaches, insomnia, and hypertension. Hold here for a few breaths and feel your partner sinking more deeply into a relaxed state.

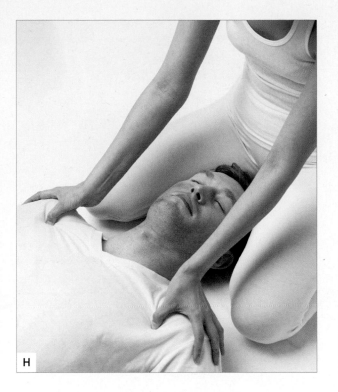

H

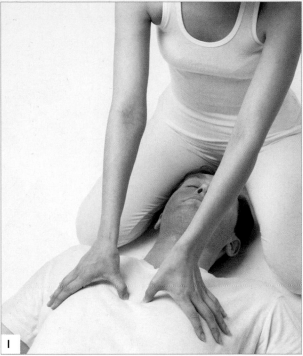

I

Press Points along the Collarbone and Sternum

Remaining at your partner's head, use finger pressure across his chest from just lateral to his sternum immediately below the collarbone and out to his shoulder (photo H). The first point you will press is called Elegant Mansion, which is thought to benefit the kidneys and lungs, and to relieve anxiety and hiccups. As you move laterally, you will press a stomach point and come to Letting Go, a lung point in the hollow below the lateral collarbone that is believed to strengthen the lungs and relieve asthma, irritability, and fatigue. Using both thumbs, return to the center of his chest and very gently press points all the way down his sternum, along the kidney meridian, potentially strengthening the urinary system (photo I).

Warning!
Avoid Shiatsu under These Conditions

Do not give a shiatsu massage to a person who has the following condition:

- Has an infectious skin disease, rash, inflamed skin, or unhealed wounds
- Is within weeks post- surgery, chemotherapy, or radiation treatments
- Has weak, previously dislocated, recently fractured, or osteoporotic bones
- Has bruises, tumors, varicose veins, a tendency toward blood clots, or a hernia

Also, on a pregnant woman who has been cleared by her physician to receive shiatsu, avoid thumbing or applying any pointed pressure below the knees, on the tops of the shoulders, and on the web of the thumbs.

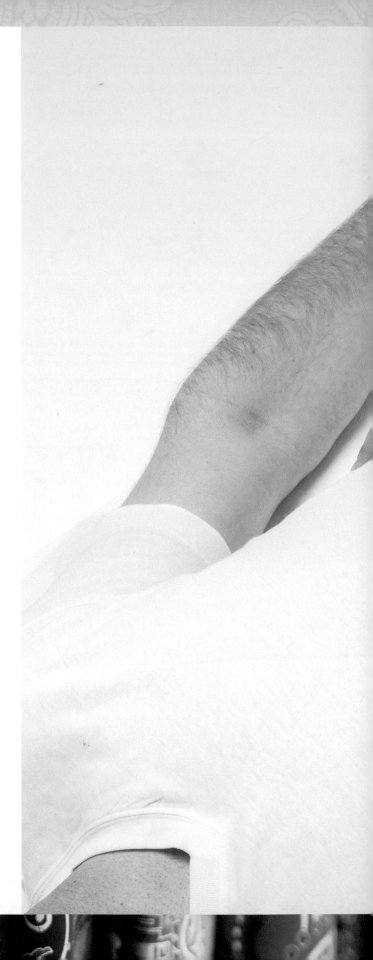

Stimulate the Lung Meridian

Kneel at your partner's right side and thumb under the edge of his rib cage, moving from the middle out to the lateral ribs, exercising caution to ease in slowly with each exhalation as he may be ticklish along the ribcage (**photo J**). Following the lower ribcage you will stimulate points on the lung meridian, with respiratory benefits, and at the point of the ribs directly below the nipples you will press a point on the spleen meridian called Abdominal Sorrow, which may provide relief for abdominal cramping, nausea, and indigestion. Once you have reached the lateral edge of the ribcage, thumb back along the line to the center.

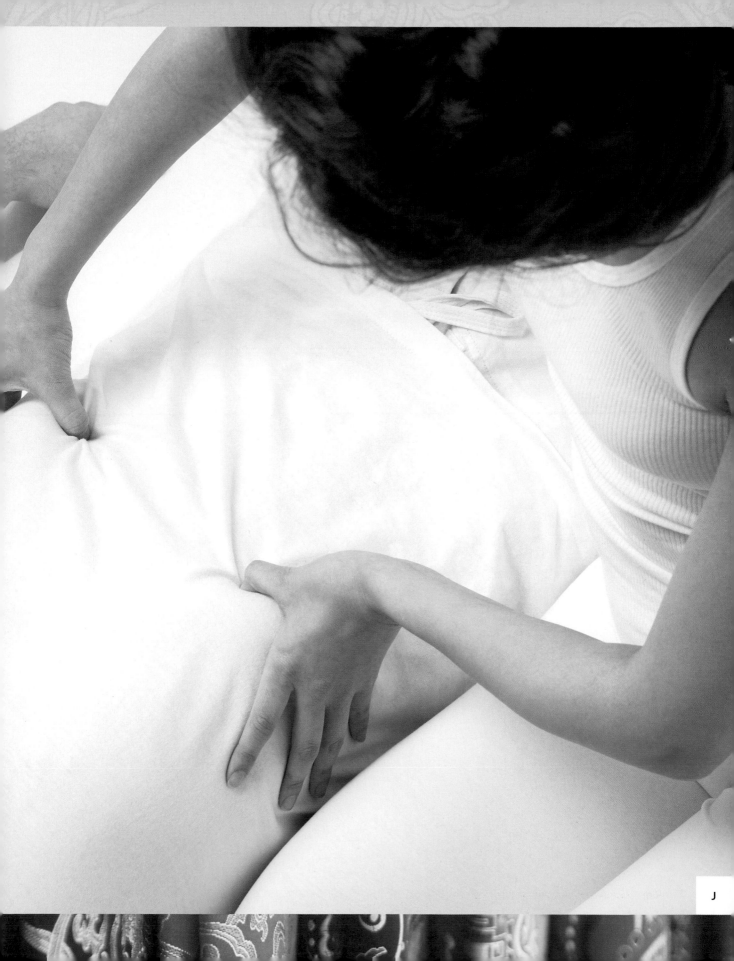

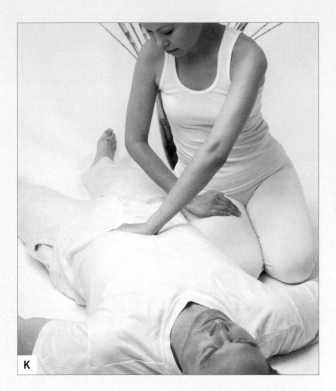

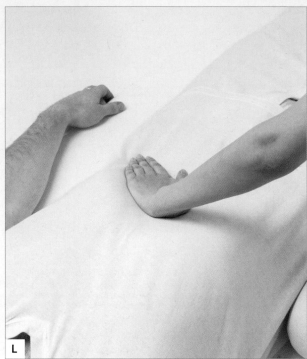

Palm the Hara

With continued caution due to the sensitivity of the abdominal area, place your palm on your partner's left abdomen with the lateral edge of your hand next to his ribcage, fingers pointing toward his right hip. You will be addressing a large primary energy center, the hara, compressing all four corners of the abdomen and below the navel, moving in a clockwise direction. The hara contains large energy areas for essentially all of the body systems, so you may consider this a full-body energy-balancing technique.

Wait for his inhalation and on the next exhale, lean your weight slightly into your palm. Hold the pressure steady on each inhalation and sink in slightly on each exhalation, for three or four rounds of breath. Then move your hand to just below his left ribcage, fingers toward his right armpit, and repeat the palming compression you performed on the other side (photo K). The next position is with your hand along the front edge of the hip bone (ilium) with your fingers pointing toward his groin (photo L) and is then mirrored on the other side of his lower abdomen (photo M), allowing your palm to sink slightly with each exhalation. Place your palm just below his navel and repeat the process there (photo N).

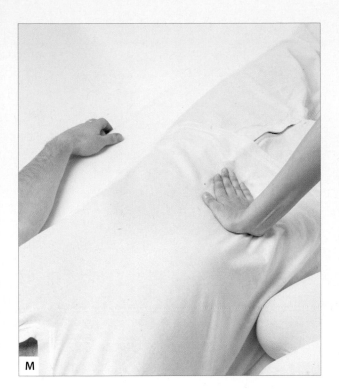

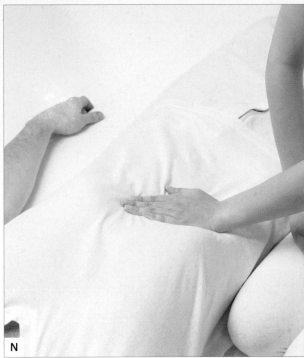

Sink into the Chest

Holding your partner's right hand in your own, lift it so that his lower arm is perpendicular with the mat and his upper arm is raised slightly off the mat. With your left palm, compress his upper chest muscle (pectoralis) with one or two hand positions, sinking in for a few breaths.

Warning! Back Off a Strong Pulse

If you feel a strong pulse in any position, reduce your pressure until you no longer feel the pulse.

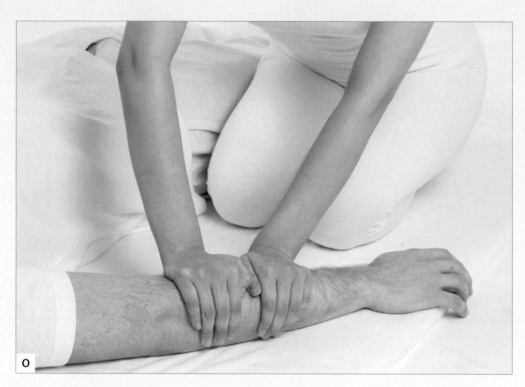

O

Points of Interest

- A point on the heart meridian at the pinky side of the wrist crease, called Spirit Gate, is beneficial for insomnia and overexcitement. Compressing it also strengthens the heart and the spirit.
- Points on the forearm pericardium at the palm just below the index finger and the middle of the wrist crease are useful for reducing fever.
- A point on the forearm three finger widths from the middle of the wrist is useful for morning sickness, motion sickness, and other types of nausea.

3. PALM AND THUMB THE ARM AND HAND

Still in the same position, continue palming your partner's upper arm (biceps) muscle, moving down to the elbow and returning all the way to his central chest. Repeat using a C hold to compress the meridians on each side of the biceps muscle.

Place your partner's arm to the side on the mat. First palm from his elbow to his palm and back to his elbow. Thumb from his elbow down the radial (thumb) side of his arm, all the way to the tip of the thumb on the lung meridian, and return palming up to the elbow. Repeat the same process to the index finger and back (spleen meridian) and to the ring finger (liver meridian) and back. Taking each side of his hand in your hands, with his palm facing down, stretch his arm alternately with one hand and then the other and then fold the sides of his hand toward his palm and open the palm.

Place his hand and arm on the mat, palm down, and palm his arm all the way up to the shoulder and back with both hands (photo O); follow this by thumbing at the ring finger to the point of his shoulder on the triple-warmer meridian (photo P). You will be addressing points on the meridian that are thought to relieve wrist, elbow, and shoulder pain as well as tendonitis, allergies, and tension.

Move to your partner's left side and repeat the sequence from palming the chest through the arm and hand.

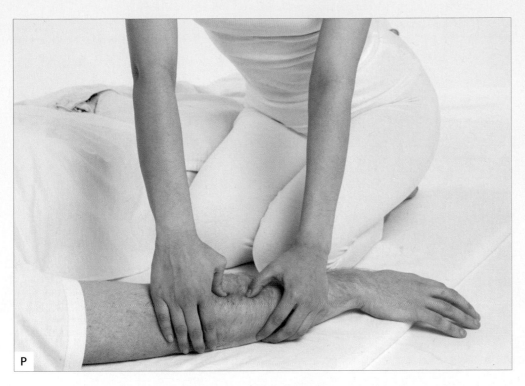

P

Better Physical, Mental, and Spiritual Health

Compressing long portions of the lung, pericardium, spleen, and heart meridians balances energy in each of those systems, resulting in relief from anxiety and emotional intensity, regulating the heart and strengthening the spirit.

4. FIND THE RANGE OF MOTION IN THE FOOT

While seated or kneeling at your partner's feet, palm the soles of his feet, pressing them outward. Perform circular friction on the anterior ankles and dorsiflex (press the ball of the foot toward the head) and plantarflex (press the sole of the foot toward the mat) the ankle.

Squeeze both sides of your partner's right foot in the same way you worked his hand in the preceding sequence, putting his ankle through all of its motions, holding his heel in your right hand and using your left to move the front of his foot, and then pulling first one side of his foot and then the other side toward you, grasping it strongly. Thumb the meridian lines on the top, or dorsal, surface of his foot in the same way the Thai sen lines in chapter 3 are thumbed. Some of the benefits of working the top of the foot include stimulating the liver point, called Bigger Rushing, for relief from hangovers and congestion and to invigorate as you thumb toward the ankle from the big toe. Above Tears—a point on the gall bladder meridian about three finger widths up the top of the foot toward the ankle from the intersection of the little toe and the fourth toe—reduces water retention and helps with sciatica and headaches. Repeat on your partner's left foot.

Of Waste and Want

The gall bladder, liver, kidney, spleen, and stomach meridians are on the anterior leg and cross the front of the ankle. You are balancing the energy in systems of the body that are involved in elimination and reproduction when you address the feet and legs. You may also relieve sciatica and headaches by stimulating the gall bladder meridian.

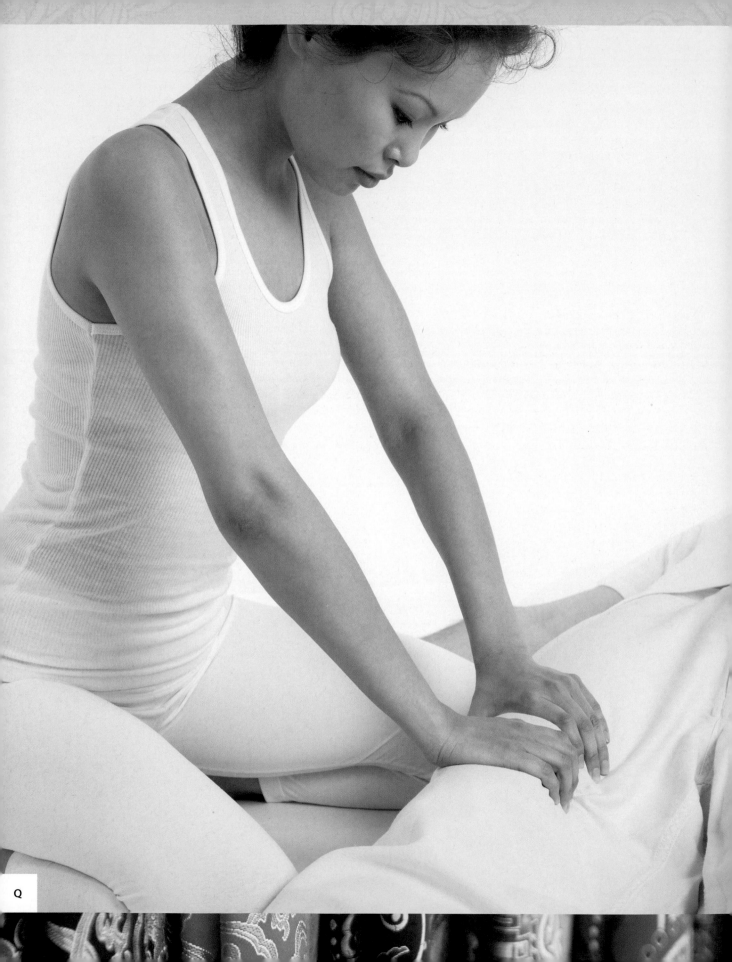

5. PALM AND THUMB THE LEG

Move to your partner's left side and starting at the ankle, palm the left leg and thigh, leaning into compressions. Then use both hands in C holds to simultaneously compress the gall bladder meridian on the lateral side and the stomach meridian on the medial side. Using your thumbs on the lateral leg, lean in and thumb to his knee and back to his ankle, rocking into the points on the gallbladder meridian.

Remaining on the left side, palm from his knee to his groin and back; then repeat the pattern with C holds along his thigh and return, rocking forward with each compression (**photo Q**). Bring his knee out to the side, with his left foot near his right knee. Place a cushion under his knee if it does not rest on the mat. Use flat hands to palm along his inner thigh from his knee to his groin and back. Be careful, especially near the knee, as the medial thigh can be tender (**photo R**).

Rotate his knee upward, placing your left knee to keep his foot from sliding, and rock his knee away from you, palming his lateral thigh along the gall bladder meridian all the way up into the hip area. Lean in, not letting his thigh come fully back to upright when you release the compressions but gradually urging it farther away from you into a greater stretch. You may also thumb up and down the thigh in this position. This work opens the posterior hip and can relieve hip pain as well as increase mobility.

Pull the Heel and Leg

Extend your partner's left leg and move to his foot, holding it at the ankle and heel, and lean back, giving traction to the whole leg and thigh for a few breaths. This is a nice reverse of the compressive weight our legs and feet carry. Place his leg back on the mat and repeat all of these actions on his right leg and thigh.

Depending on your partner's size relative to your own and his flexibility, you may then lift his extended legs, stretching them upward as you do so to a position where the soles of his feet are toward the ceiling, and hold for a few breaths. This will stretch the length of the bladder meridian and begin to loosen tight hamstring muscles.

Magnificent Points

Points stimulated along this meridian may relieve ankle and low back pain, including sciatica. At mid-calf is a point called Supporting Mountain, which is said to relieve cramps, low back pain, leg pain, and swelling. Above it, behind the knee, is a point called Commanding Activity, which may strengthen the lower back and knees and assist with back pain and knee stiffness.

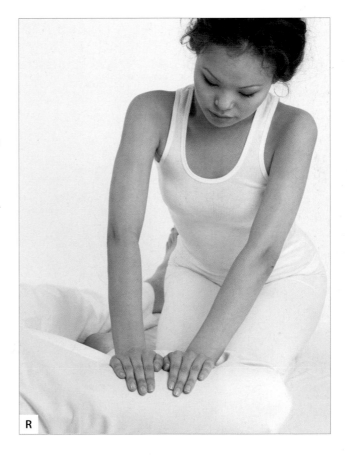

R

6. TRANSITION TO PRONE FOR BACK AND SHOULDERS

Have your partner turn to face down, using a face cradle or rolled towel to keep his neck in a neutral position. You can use a pillow under his chest if it makes him more comfortable. Kneel with one knee between his legs and your other foot flat on the mat next to his hip. Alternating hands or pressing with both hands at once, palm from his waistline to his shoulders, then back down to the sacrum. Then thumb along the ridge of muscle about 1 inch (2.5 cm) lateral to his spine from his waistline to his shoulders and back down, repeating the thumb about 3 inches (7.6 cm) lateral to his spine.

Palm and Thumb the Back and Buttock

Moving to your partner's left side, kneel and rock into palming compressions on the right side of his back, alternating your hands from his waistline to his shoulder and back to his hip; then thumb along the same line, sinking in and then pressing away from the pronounced band of muscles close to his spine using both thumbs at once on each exhalation (photo S). Alternately, you may lean your elbows into the muscle and sink straight into it, working up to the shoulder and back.

Leaning forward with your shoulders over your hands, palm along your partner's buttock, or gluteal muscles, and out to his hip. Kneel on your left knee and place your right foot on the mat just beyond his right hip. Thumb lines starting from the top of his sacrum out to his hip, each time starting lower on the sacrum. Palm the gluteal area again after you thumb lines in the same direction (out to the hip) and continue palming right above this crest of the hip, moving from just lateral to the spine and out to the edge of the waistline.

If you feel comfortable in this position, you can turn your arm parallel to his spine and press just lateral to his spine on the right side of his back. Move to his right side and repeat these two sequences.

Warning! Increase Pressure Gradually

The muscle here, called quadratus lumborum, is a big player in low back pain and may be tender, so only gradually increase the pressure with which you are leaning into it.

Pointed Relief for "Pain in the Butt"

Working the gall bladder point called Jumping Circle, a point midway between the sacrum and the hip near the middle of the buttock, may relieve irritation and frustration.

Overworked Erector

The muscles running parallel to the spine, the erector spinae, work overtime to maintain our upright position, whether seated or standing, so they frequently need targeted massage. The extra work is worth it, as the associated meridian includes points for other meridians.

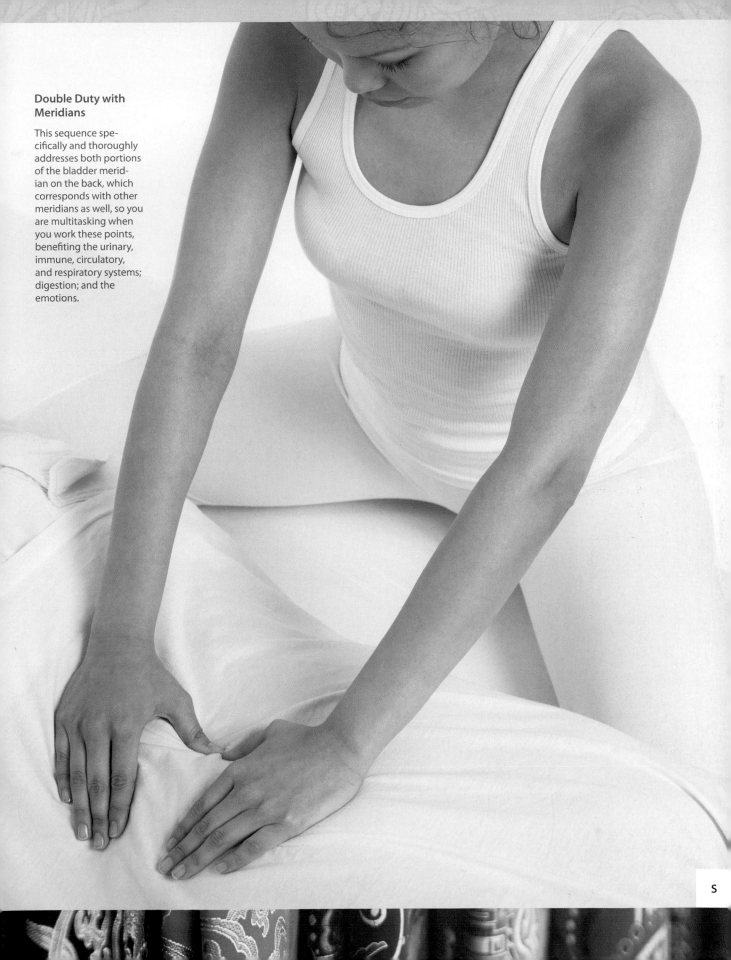

Double Duty with Meridians

This sequence specifically and thoroughly addresses both portions of the bladder meridian on the back, which corresponds with other meridians as well, so you are multitasking when you work these points, benefiting the urinary, immune, circulatory, and respiratory systems; digestion; and the emotions.

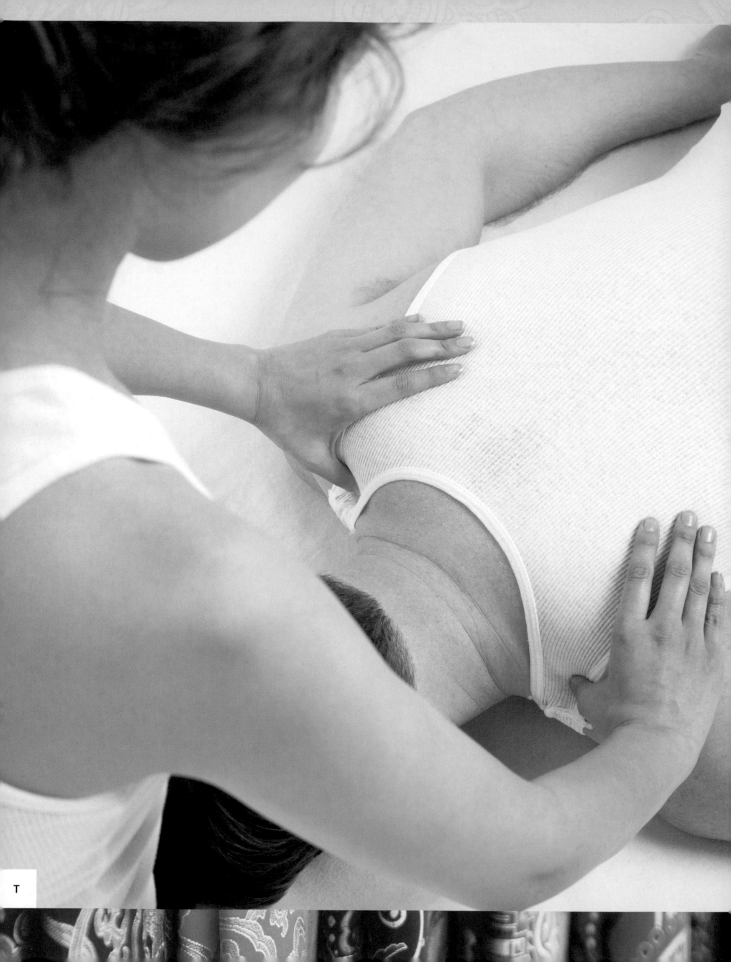

Press and Hold the Sacrum

With your thumbs, press and hold the indentations all over your partner's sacrum. These sacral points can relieve pelvis discomfort, whether from labor, menstruation, or sciatica, and may strengthen reproductive organs.

Move to Shoulder

Kneel or sit with your knees apart at your partner's head. Lean in and thumb right above his shoulder blade, or scapula, from the shoulder joint to the base of the neck (**photo T**). Traditionally, this is done with one hand, with the other hand resting on the opposite shoulder, but you may choose to thumb both sides at once. Then thumb the middle of your partner's scapula and lean the side of your hand(s) at the crease above the posterior armpit. All of these points are on the small intestine meridian and are effective for relief of tension and discomfort in the neck and shoulders.

From Triceps to Pinky

Move to your partner's left side, moving his upper arm out to the side and away from his torso, and support his forearm with your right hand while you palm the back of his arm (triceps muscle) to his wrist and back up to his shoulder. As you palm his triceps, press in from the lower portion of his arm rather than straight down. This will generally address the small intestine and heart meridians. You may thumb the heart and pericardium meridians all the way down to the end of the little finger and middle finger. Repeat on the right side.

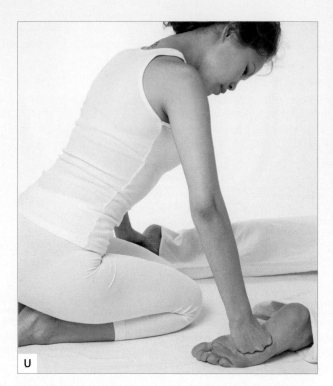

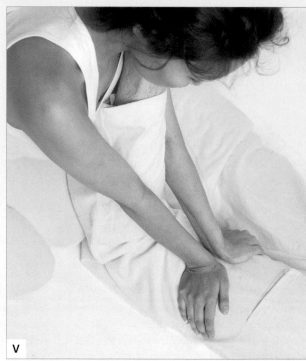

7. ROCK THE FEET AND BACK OF THE LEGS

Kneel between your partner's legs and place your fists on the soles of his feet, rocking back and forth on them several times **(photo U)**. Alternately, you may stand facing his head and gently walk along the medial arch from the front of his heels to the balls of his feet, alternating your weight from one foot to the other. All of these actions will stimulate kidney points on the foot, calming restlessness and possibly alleviating headaches and nosebleeds.

Use flat hands to palm the back of his leg and thigh, starting at his ankle. Palm up to his upper thigh and return to his ankles for the bladder meridian; then repeat the process with the C hold, simulating the kidney, gall bladder, and liver meridians. This provides such possible benefits as reducing knee and other joint pain and stiffness, as well as relieving edema, swelling, water retention, and constipation.

Return to kneeling at the right of your partner and thumb from his ankle, up the center of his leg and thigh, and returning to his ankle along the bladder meridian. You may find it useful to have your right knee next to his right thigh and your left foot on the mat lateral to his left knee.

Move to a kneeling position next to his right hip and place his anterior ankle on your shoulder. Palm the back of his thigh (hamstrings) from above his knee to the top of his thigh and back to his knee **(photo V)**, first with a C hold and then with a flat palm, and finally thumb the bladder meridian on the same pathway. Palming and thumbing on the posterior thigh with the hamstrings relaxed can help release tightness that can contribute to low back pain.

Warning!

Don't Try This on Problematic Knees

If your partner has any knee problems, you may want to leave this next sequence out. Before returning your partner's lower leg to the mat, use both hands on his foot to swing his knee from side to side. Then, when his knee is away from his torso, use your hand on the sole of his foot to bring his knee as close to perpendicular to his body as possible, with his right foot toward his left knee. First palm and then thumb from the lateral side of his foot, up his calf and thigh, to his hip, and then back to his ankle. You will be addressing the gall bladder meridian, including points on the foot and in front of the ankle bone that may help with shoulder and side pain, ankle sprains, and arthritic pain. At the lateral knee, a point called Sunny Side of the Mountain may reduce knee pain and relax the lower body muscles.

At the most lateral point of the hip, Jumping Circle may reduce hip pain and improve joint mobility as well as moderate frustration and irritation. Extend your partner's leg as you return it to the mat and kneel at his left side, repeating the actions you have completed on the right side.

Still kneeling on the left side, with your right hand on the front of your partner's right ankle, flex his knee so that his heel comes toward his buttocks. Your left hand will be pressing down on the sacrum and toward his feet to keep his hips from lifting and to lengthen his back. Hold for a few breaths and then return his right knee to the mat and repeat with his left leg, then with both legs simultaneously. This move stretches along the stomach, spleen, and liver meridians, toning and balancing them. Return your partner to a supine position.

Finishing Shiatsu

Go to your partner's feet. Holding his ankles, lift his legs about 1 foot (30.5 cm) off the mat and lean back to create some traction for his legs, hips, and lower back. Bring his legs up higher but not past ninety degrees, stretching the bladder meridian again. Push up using your legs rather than your back to assist in the stretch, particularly if you are smaller than your partner.

Take your partner's legs farther over, if possible, and as his hips lift, support them with your legs just below your knees. If your partner has no cervical spine (neck) issues, you may place the soles of his feet together, asking him to allow his knees to relax out to the sides. Ideally, you should be able to look down through his arches and see his face. This stretch can relax the lower back and

hips after they are warmed up from the rest of the session and will stretch along the kidney and bladder meridians. Bring his knees together and press them toward his chest. Hold and take a few breaths. Bring his feet to the mat and then slide his legs to extend them on the mat, supporting them under the knees all the way down.

Repeat some of the sequence you performed on your partner's neck, as it may have tightened up some during the other sequences and particularly from lying face down. End with a closing hold on his shoulders or the heart while seated at his head, or move to his left side and place your left hand on his forehead and your right hand on his hara or heart. Take several breaths and then take your hands away very slowly.

Shiatsu in a Seat

It is possible to do shiatsu on a seated partner, either in a chair or on the mat. If you wish to integrate a seated portion to this routine, see chapter 4 on Thai massage; the seated section is very close to a shiatsu seated sequence.

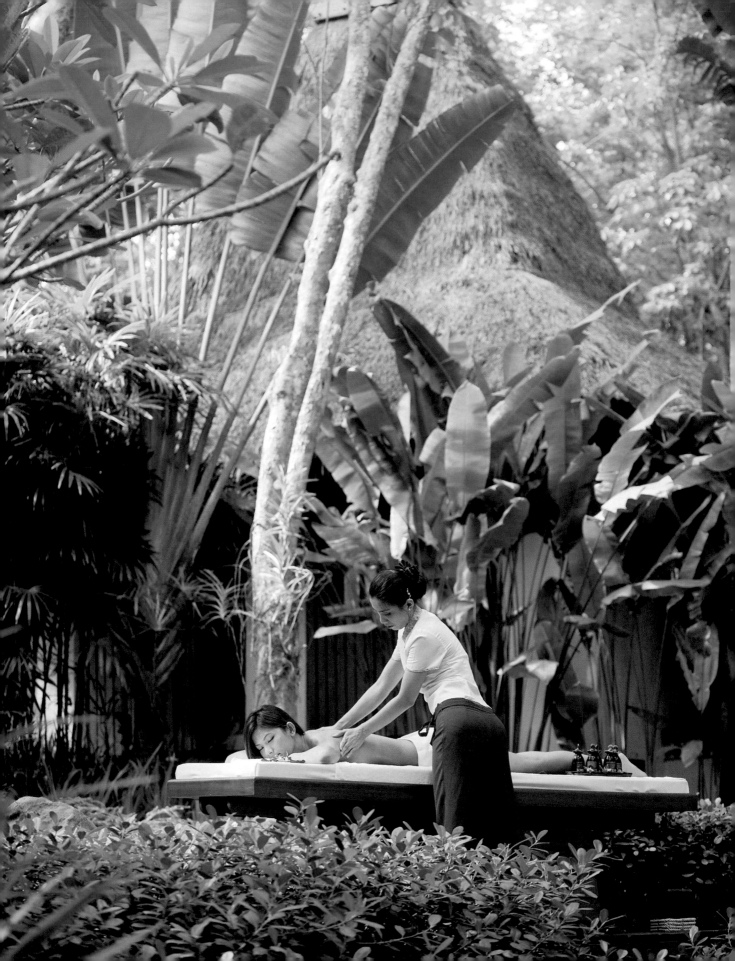

CHAPTER 9

Understanding Basic Theory and Practice

When applying any type of massage stroke, begin superficially, or close to the surface, and gradually sink in deeper as you perform repetitions. This gives the body an opportunity to warm up and allow deeper access as both the receiver and the particular muscle accept increasing depth of strokes. Start with broad strokes, generally using the whole hand or forearm, and gradually work more specifically, using fingers. This also allows the tissue to warm up and accept smaller and more targeted pressure.

In general, apply between three and six strokes to give your partner a chance to relax into what you're doing without becoming annoyed by it. Using more than ten strokes of the same kind would probably irritate her.

Massage Strokes

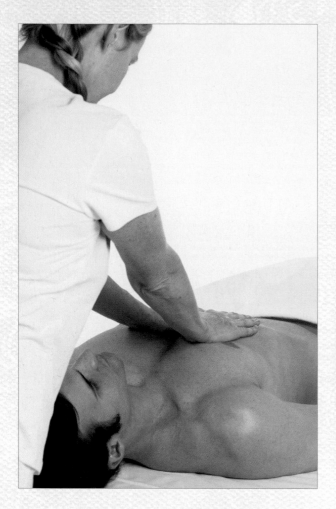

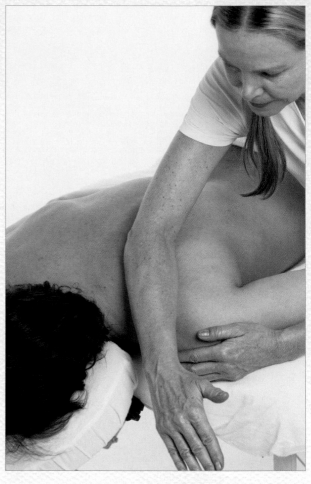

Effleurage—using the flat palm with fingers together, you glide away from your torso with neutral (not flexed or hyperextended) wrists. Effleurage strokes may be performed with one or both hands, or with forearms in some areas of the body

**Warning!
Mind Your Elbows**

Don't use your elbows unless you are a seasoned professional; it's just too easy to hurt your partner. Also, do not press directly and strongly on any bones, especially the spinous processes of the vertebral column, the part of the spine you can feel on the back.

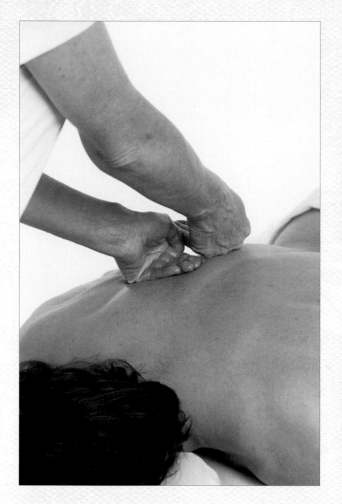
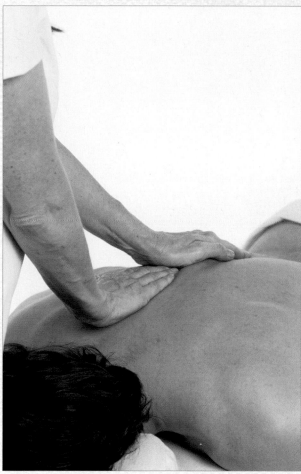

Pushing strokes—Alternating effleurage with the backs of fingers and the palms

Massage Strokes *(cont.)*

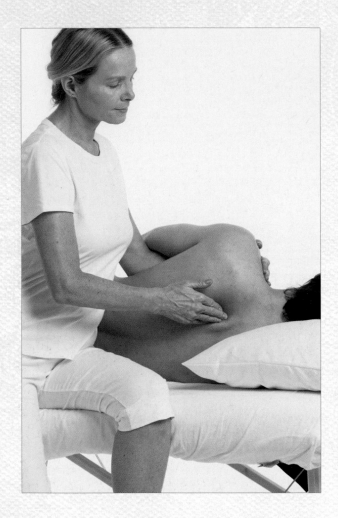

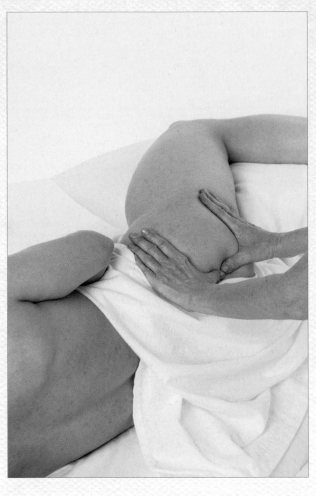

Friction—Small circles or short back-and-forth movements applied with the fingers

Stripping—Short friction strokes applied unidirectionally

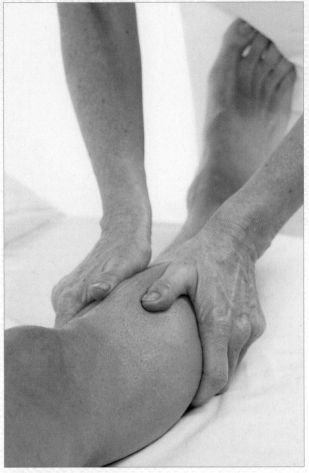

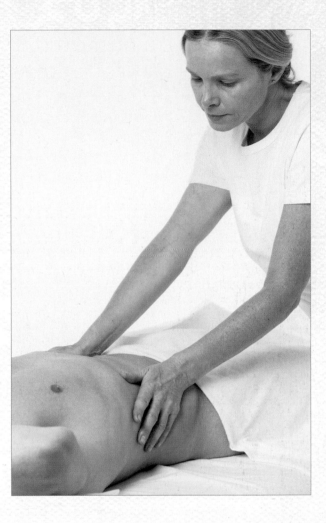

Petrissage—Kneading, lifting, and squeezing muscle tissue with the palm in full contact with the skin

Spreading—A type of effleurage stroke in which the hands move apart to stretch the skin and underlying muscles

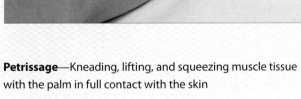

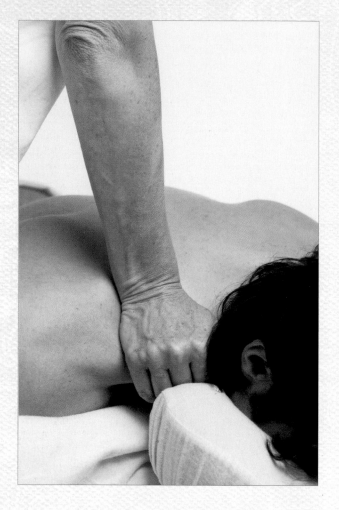

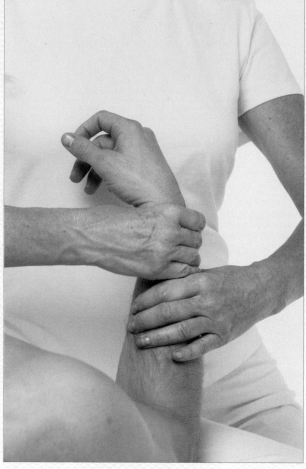

Compression—Pressing downward into the tissue with fingers, thumbs, or forearm, or sqeezing the tissue with static pressure between fingers and heel of hand

Wringing—Grasping an area, usually of a limb, and working your hands in opposition to each other, as if wringing water out of a towel

Tapotement (right)—Brisk percussive movements performed in a rapid, rhythmic fashion

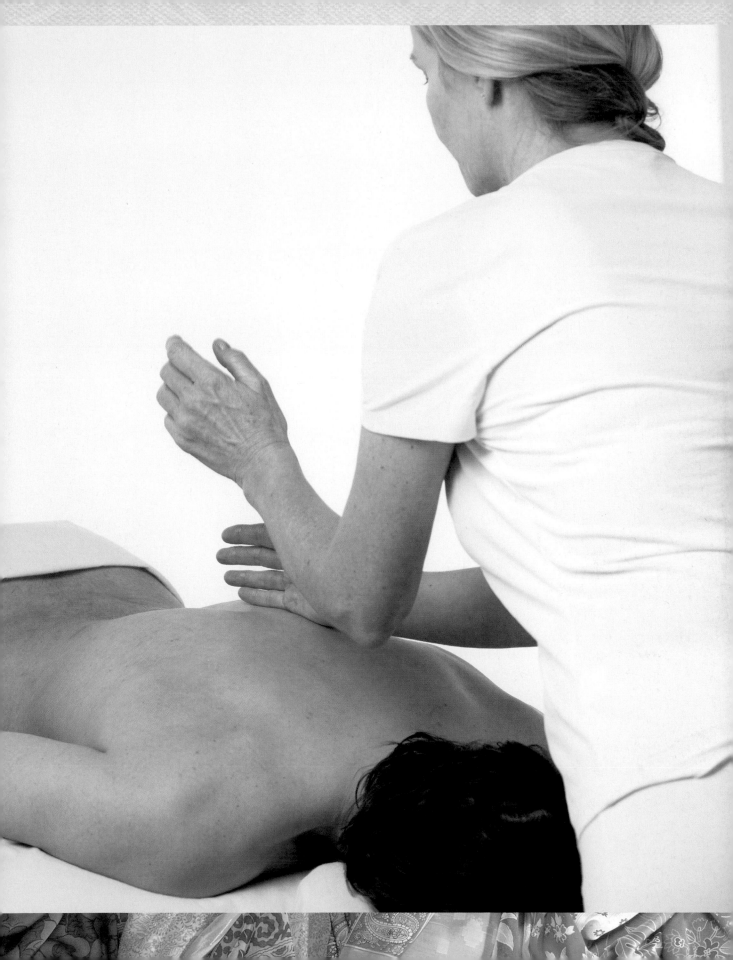

DIFFERENTIATE BETWEEN DEPTH AND PRESSURE

There is a difference between depth and pressure. Many techniques that use stretching or energy manipulation can have a very deep and therapeutic effect without the application of a lot of pressure. Massaging with finesse rather than force is generally preferable, for both the giver and the receiver. In all forms of massage, it is preferable to use gradual penetration into deeper layers of the body, waiting for the tissue to "invite" you in. Pushing through resistance is often painful and can cause lingering discomfort and injury. The deeper you intend to work, the slower you must perform compressions or strokes, or the body will resist and the receiver will experience pain.

If you feel a strong pulse under your fingers or hand, especially at the neck, groin, or abdomen, you have two choices: Lighten your pressure until you do not feel the pulse or move your hand to a location where the pulse is not present. When massaging slim, narrow-hipped people, you may find there is nowhere on the abdomen you do not feel a strong pulse; go lightly or skip the abdominal massage.

When performing range-of-motion techniques, feel for end points, or points where the movement slows and meets restriction. It is imperative that you move a limb or other area of the body through its range of motion very slowly, as it is difficult to detect "end feel" when you are moving the body too quickly, and you can exceed the comfortable and normal range before you are aware you have reached the joint's limitation. You should seek to encourage a limb to very gradually move a little farther into its range of motion, rather than apply any force. When in doubt, slow is always preferable to fast when it comes to bodywork, although if your partner is preparing for an athletic event, doing faster massage will have a stimulating preparatory effect.

JUDGE HOLDS AND REPETITIONS BY RESPONSE

There are some guidelines for how long to hold compressions, mostly in terms of the approximate number of breaths, but what is most important is that you focus on your partner's response to what you are doing and respond to that rather than go through some arbitrary rote routine. That being said, avoid repeating a stroke more than a dozen times, as it can become tedious and irritating; also avoid changing strokes before your partner's nervous system has a chance to relax into what's happening. Somewhere around three to five repetitions of most strokes is ideal, although you may find areas of your partner's body where it just feels right to perform more or less.

Anatomical and Directional Terms

In this section, you'll find a helpful review of directional terms as well as diagrams showing the locations of many of the muscles and bones discussed in the step-by-step techniques described in this book. You will find the definitions of additional terms in the Glossary section, beginning on page 235.

Anterior—Front of the body

Posterior—Back of the body

Dorsal—Back of the hand, forearm, or foot

Ventral—Palm of the hand, sole of the foot

Lateral—A relational term; farther from the midline of the body

Medial—A relational term; closer to the midline of the body

Superior—A relational term; closer to the top of the body, or the head

Inferior—A relational term; closer to the bottom of the body, or the feet)

Supine—Face up

Prone—Face down

Supinated—Palms facing up

Pronated—Palms facing down

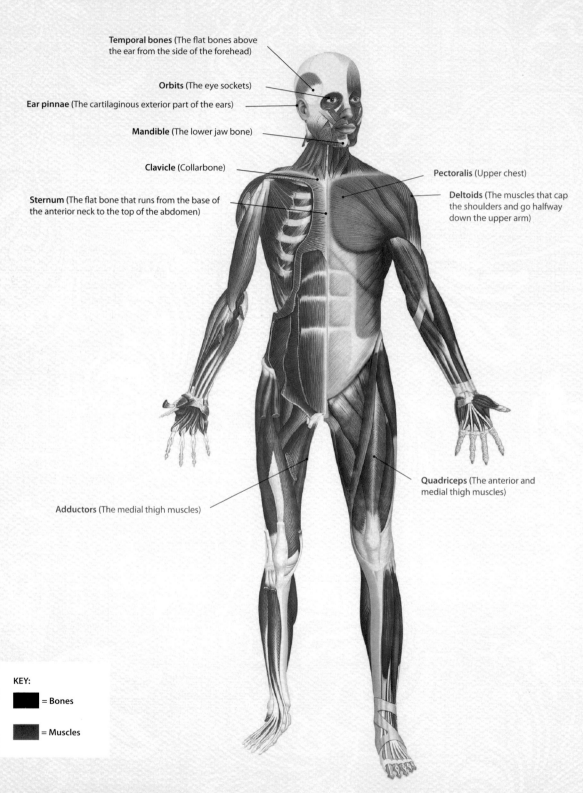

Temporal bones (The flat bones above the ear from the side of the forehead)

Orbits (The eye sockets)

Ear pinnae (The cartilaginous exterior part of the ears)

Mandible (The lower jaw bone)

Clavicle (Collarbone)

Sternum (The flat bone that runs from the base of the anterior neck to the top of the abdomen)

Pectoralis (Upper chest)

Deltoids (The muscles that cap the shoulders and go halfway down the upper arm)

Quadriceps (The anterior and medial thigh muscles)

Adductors (The medial thigh muscles)

KEY:

■ = Bones

■ = Muscles

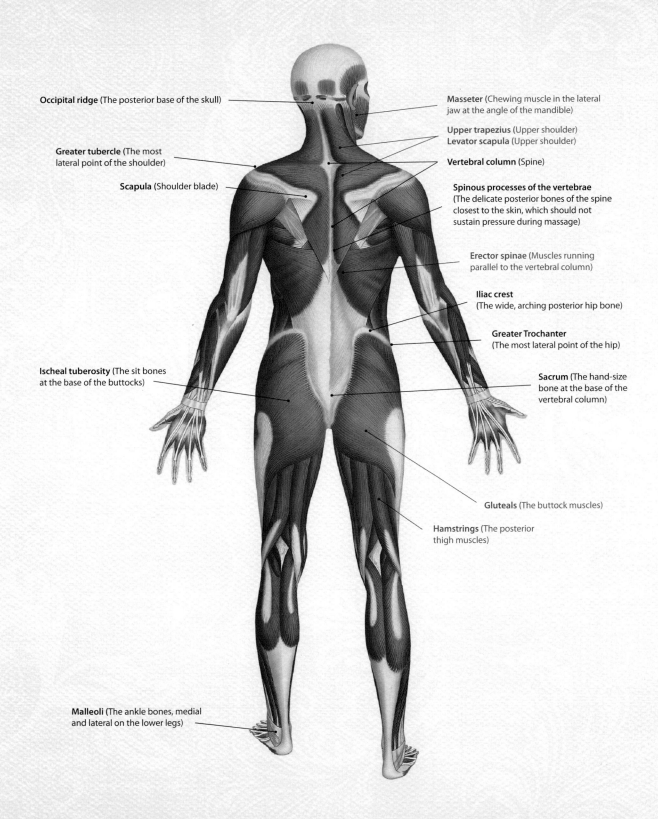

Occipital ridge (The posterior base of the skull)

Masseter (Chewing muscle in the lateral jaw at the angle of the mandible)

Upper trapezius (Upper shoulder)
Levator scapula (Upper shoulder)

Greater tubercle (The most lateral point of the shoulder)

Vertebral column (Spine)

Scapula (Shoulder blade)

Spinous processes of the vertebrae (The delicate posterior bones of the spine closest to the skin, which should not sustain pressure during massage)

Erector spinae (Muscles running parallel to the vertebral column)

Iliac crest (The wide, arching posterior hip bone)

Greater Trochanter (The most lateral point of the hip)

Ischeal tuberosity (The sit bones at the base of the buttocks)

Sacrum (The hand-size bone at the base of the vertebral column)

Gluteals (The buttock muscles)

Hamstrings (The posterior thigh muscles)

Malleoli (The ankle bones, medial and lateral on the lower legs)

The Massage Environment: Maximum Comfort

Maximum comfort is key for massage to be pleasant and effective for relaxation and stress relief. Your partner should feel comfortable, at ease, and secure in the room you chose for massage. A small room is both cozy and easier to heat, although your room choice will be limited by the amount of space available to you. Generally, a room between 72°F and 74°F (22°C and 23°C) will provide enough warmth for the receiver while not overheating the active giver too much. Covering is useful for all forms of massage. Some forms of massage, such as Swedish, hot stone, and lomi lomi, require direct access to the skin, so draping with a sheet or bath towel provides comfort. Cotton or cotton flannel sheets are preferable to synthetic fabric blends. Other forms such as shiatsu, Thai, Tantsu, and polarity are generally performed on a clothed receiver, who should be dressed in comfortable, loose, preferably cotton garments.

Seek a Medical Release for These Conditions

People with the following health conditions should seek a medical release before receiving massage:

- Heart disease and circulatory conditions such as uncontrolled high blood pressure, aortic aneurism, and a tendency to have blood clots (thrombosis)—Avoid pressure on varicose veins.
- Liver or kidney diseases that put a strain on the whole system
- Systemic infections such as colds, flu, and blood poisoning.
- Autoimmune disorders such as lupus, rheumatoid arthritis, and multiple sclerosis
- Osteoporosis, recent fractures, dislocations, joint conditions, and bone diseases.
- Infectious skin disease, rash, or open wounds

Pregnant women and people who have just undergone surgery, chemotherapy, or radiation should also check with their doctors before receiving bodywork. In addition, care must be exercised when massaging a person who has sensory impairment or is under the influence of drugs—either prescription or recreational—that might compromise her ability to sense whether pressure, heat, or stretch is too intense and advise you of that fact.

Your own clothing should be loose enough to allow you to move freely but not so loose that it drags across your partner's body. Likewise, your hair should be out of the way so that you don't have to keep sweeping it from your face and pulled back so that it does not touch your partner's body. If you tend to sweat when you are exerting yourself, having a hand towel nearby to wipe your face or wearing a headband to catch perspiration before it drips onto your partner will be helpful. Massage is a very physical activity, and the room you will massage in should be warm.

LOW LIGHT AND MUSIC

Indirect, low lighting or natural filtered sunlight is more relaxing than bright overhead lights; such lighting creates a more serene mood and it won't be shining in your partner's eyes when she is face up (supine). If your partner lacks body confidence, low lighting can be reassuring. Candles can produce an inviting and intimate environment. Quiet, soothing music is a pleasant addition to massage, but you may want to make sure you key into the rhythm of your partner's breath rather than the music's rhythm for some modalities, such as Thai and Tantsu. Lomi lomi, being vigorous and faster-paced, lends itself to somewhat faster music with a pronounced beat (or Hawaiian music, which will remind you to hula!), while the relaxation in Swedish and hot stone massages is enhanced by slow music.

FURNITURE, MATS, CUSHIONS, AND CRADLES

Create a space for massage where you can have room to spread out. Whether you are using a massage table or a mat, it is useful to have at least 3 feet (91.4 cm) of space around the perimeter for a chair, stool, or cushion and room to extend your own body when necessary to avoid awkward positioning. You may not have space in your home to devote a full-time area to massage, so a folding portable massage table or floor mat will serve you

well. When selecting a massage table, make sure it is sturdy and is rated for the heaviest person you will likely massage, including your own weight if you are likely to get up on the table to perform some actions, as in the table adaptations for Thai massage. Folding massage tables set up quickly and are easily carried and stored in a closet or under the bed.

A regular chair or stool works well for portions of a table massage when you will be seated to massage your partner's head, face, and neck or feet. Experiment with different heights by adding a cushion to the seat of a chair that feels too low, for instance.

Mats are very portable and usually roll to a smaller size than a massage table for storage. A mat should be at least 60" x 80" (1.5 x 2 m) and may include a supplemental kneeling pad; if it doesn't, you can substitute a flat cushion. Mats marketed primarily for Thai massage work fine for all the mat-based techniques in this book. You can use a sheet or blanket to cover the mat surface for massage or purchase a mat with a removable cover; otherwise, the mat will become unpleasant after much use. (You can find sources for massage tables and floor mats in the Resources section at the end of this book.) Have a few cushions close at hand for massage on a table or a floor mat. A cushion to bolster your partner's knees when she is in the face-up (supine) position takes pressure off her lower back. A cushion under her ankles when she is face down makes her ankles and calves more comfortable. A cushion under her head when she is lying on her side and another for between her knees and ankles will keep her joints neutral and padded; an additional cushion to support her upper arm is also helpful. Some individuals get congested when laying flat on their back, so a cushion under your partner's head when she is in the supine position is welcome.

A face cradle or towel rolled to simulate a face cradle is essential for face-down or prone massage. Traditionally, people just turned their heads to the left or right, but it is much more comfortable to have the neck in a neutral position and safer for the person receiving the massage. Most massage tables come with a face cradle, and one floor-mat system includes a face cradle for floor use.

LUBRICANTS VARY BY TECHNIQUE

Lomi lomi is the "juiciest" modality in this book and traditionally requires a generous application of oil, while Swedish massage is best done with more sparing use of lubricant, and hot stone massage requires a moderate amount of lubricant. The purpose of a lubricant is to reduce friction on the skin, allowing your hands or stones to glide.

Lubricants can be liquid in the form of lotions, creams, or oils, either commercial products or simple vegetable oil. Some people are allergic to nut oils; peanut oil and coconut oils are particularly allergenic. If your partner is not sensitive to nuts, almond oil is a nice choice. Baby oil is mineral oil, which clogs pores and strips fat-soluble vitamins from the body, so avoid using it. Professional-quality lubricants in cream or lotion form have the benefit of better absorption than oil, with similar workability.

Besides the oil and corn starch found at grocery stores, you can find lubricants in health food stores, drugstores, and cosmetic supply shops. Professional massage lubricants can be ordered from suppliers listed in the Resources section, and you may want to find out from a local massage therapist or massage school what brands and formulations they use. Many companies are offering natural and organic lubricants in response to demand for these products.

Even though in some of the massage forms detailed in this book the receiver is dressed, making lubricant unnecessary, you don't need to be a purist. You may add some lubricant on dry hands or feet as you feel will be beneficial. Your own hands need to be well maintained and smooth, with short nails; the lubricant you use for massage may be a good choice to use as a regular hand cream.

COMMUNICATION IS KEY

Never, ever assume that because you like certain massage strokes or a certain amount of pressure or pace, your partner will enjoy the same things. It is very important to receive feedback from your partner while you are performing massage. You can guess that pressure was too hard if your partner grimaces, holds her breath, or clenches her fists, but ask anyway; perhaps the stroke would be fine if you performed it more slowly. When you are receiving massage it is effective to say, "It would feel better if you did …" and then to state the change you're seeking—slower, lighter, deeper, and so forth—than to say "Ouch, that hurts!" or similar statements. Be constructive in your feedback and gracious in accepting feedback. After all, you probably would like your partner to give you more massages and ones that increasingly are in line with your preferences.

Glossary

Acupressure

Acupressure is an ancient healing art that uses the fingers to press key points on the surface of the skin to stimulate the body's natural self-healing. When these points are pressed, they release muscular tension and promote the circulation of blood and the body's life force (sometimes known as qi or chi) to aid healing.

Acute

A condition that had abrupt onset, in reference to a disease is called acute. It often also connotes an illness of short duration, that is rapidly progressive and in need of urgent care.

Adductors

This is a muscle group on the medial thigh that attaches on the pubic bone, or anterior pelvis, and the femur, responsible for moving the leg and thigh medially.

Anterior

This term refers to any area pertaining to the front of the body.

Arthritis

Inflammation of a joint or joints. When joints are inflamed, they can develop stiffness, warmth, swelling, redness, and pain and may contraindicate massage. The most common form, osteoarthritis, is a result of normal wear and tear and frequently improves as a result of massage. Many of the other forms of arthritis are autoimmune and/or inflammatory in nature, and massage is contraindicated when inflammation is present or if increasing circulation to the area might exacerbate the condition.

Asian bodywork

This form of bod work focuses on monitoring the flow of the vital life energy (known as chi, ki, prana, or qi). Using physical pressure and manipulation, the practitioner evaluates and works with this energy flow to attain a state of balance. Popular modalities include shiatsu, amna, jin shin do, Thai, and tuina.

Ayurveda

The 5,000-year-old medical system of India is called Ayurveda. It is also a philosophy that offers a variety of practices, including massage, for creating harmony and balance in life.

Bodywork

Body work is a general term for practices involving touch and movement in which the giver uses manual techniques to promote the health of the receiver. Most healing massage techniques are considered forms of bodywork.

Chi

Chi is a person's vital energy, also called qi in Asian bodywork.

Chronic

A condition that is long-standing, causing disability or discomfort for an extended period of time. The person may not even remember the injury or illness.

Clavicle

The clavicle, or the collarbone, a horizontal bone in the upper chest between the sternum and the scapula.

Compression

A compression is static, or stationary, pressure applied to an area of the body or a trigger point with the thumb, the heel of the hand, the fingertips, or sometimes the elbow. The pressure used is always within the receiver's pain tolerance, and the length of time varies—usually until the pain dissipates. Communication with the receiver is essential during compression.

Contraindication

A contraindication is a condition that would limit the benefit of massage or would make a session more harmful than healthful. Contraindications include flare-ups of autoimmune disorders, fevers, colds, systemic infections, at-risk pregnancies, and compromised major bodily systems, such as the urinary, digestive, or circulatory system, since massage would put more of a strain on an already weakened system of the body.

Deltoids

These are the large muscles that cap the shoulders and attach midway down the humerus (upper arm bone), and perform all the actions the arm can make at the shoulder joint.

Dorsal

This term refers to any area pertaining to the back of the body and is frequently used to denote the backs of the hands or feet.

Draping

This is the use of sheets, towels, or other materials to cover receivers of massage to preserve their privacy and modesty and for warmth. In professional massage therapy, practice draping is mandated to ensure appropriate professional boundaries for sessions.

Effleurage

Effleurage is a Western massage therapy technique that includes movements which glide over the body with a smooth continuous motion.

Erector spinae

This is the band of muscles that parallels the vertebral column from the iliac crest to the base of the skull, and which is responsible for maintaining the upright position of the spine.

Essential oils

Natural substances extracted from botanical sources such as grasses, flowers, herbs, trees, and spices, usually through a process called steam *distillation*. Oils can soothe, relax, rejuvenate, sedate, energize, or alleviate pain, thereby affecting the body physically, energetically, and emotionally.

Exhalation

Exhalation is the act of expelling air from the lungs.

Foot zone therapy

Based on the premise that energy flows through the body in meridians from the brain to the feet. Every organ and cell has a representative point on the foot, and when pressure is applied, the brain sends a signal to that organ. Zone therapy is related closely to reflexology.

Friction

The deepest of Swedish massage strokes. Friction uses fairly deep, circular, or cross-fiber movements applied to soft tissue, causing the underlying layers of tissue to rub against each other. This causes an increase in blood flow to the massaged area and can realign or remodel tissue.

Gluteal muscles

These are the muscles on the posterior and lateral pelvis which provide movement of the leg at the hip, with attachments on the ilium, sacrum, and trochanter.

Greater trochanter

This is a large, bony, lateral protuberance near the superior end of the femur, or upper leg bone, which forms the most lateral point of the hip.

Greater tubercle

This is a bony protuberance near the superior end of the humerus, or upper arm bone, which forms the most lateral point of the shoulder.

Hamstrings

Hamstrings are a group of muscles that attach to the sit bones (ischeal tuberosities) and cross the knee joint, with attachments on the tibia and fibula of the lower leg. These muscles flex the knee and extend the hip and are very prone to shortening, especially in athletic individuals. Having tight hamstrings can put strain on the lower back, so addressing these muscles with massage has effects on the thigh and back.

Hara

Hara is the source of health, vitality, and power and the physical center of the body. Bounded by the lower rib cage and the pelvic bowl, the hara includes all the vital organs of the body, with the exception of the heart and lungs, but even these have a reflexive, energetic presence here. In Chinese medicine, the hara is located about 1 inch (2.5 cm) below the navel and is considered to be the root of vital energy, regulating our physiological and spiritual well-being. It is seen as controlling the metabolism of the blood and organs, and producing the qi that flows along our meridians.

Healing

Healing is the process of regaining health or optimal functioning after an injury, disease, or other debilitating condition.

Hot stone

This is a massage technique used in conjunction with other modalities, in which warmed stones are placed on points, such as acupuncture points or chakras (energy centers), and are sometimes used as massage tools.

Iliac crest

This is the superior edge of the ilium, which arches from the sacrum posteriorly to the lateral hip.

Ilium

This is the large wing-like hip bone that attaches to the sacrum posteriorly, and includes the socket (the acetabulum) into which the head of the femur articulates to form the hip joint.

Inferior

Interior is a term that indicates that a place on the body is lower on the body than another place. For instance, the pelvis is inferior to the ribcage.

Inflammation

Inflammation is a basic way in which the body reacts to infection, irritation, or some other injury. The key features include redness, warmth, swelling, loss of function, and pain. Inflammation is a type of nonspecific immune response and is functional for healing in many cases.

Ingham Method

This is a form of zone therapy or reflexology. In the 1930s, Eunice Ingham, a physiotherapist, used zone therapy on patients. She mapped the entire body as reflex areas on the feet. Ingham first used this method to reduce pain, but then she enlarged the work into the Ingham Reflex Method of Compression Massage, later known as reflexology.

Inhalation

Also called inspiration, this is the intake of air into the lungs.

Joint mobilization

This is the act of moving a limb through its normal range of motion slowly and carefully, making sure you do not torque any joint by applying substantial pressure in any direction. Watch your partner's face as you move an arm or leg, and do not take the limb farther if you see even a hint of a grimace as you move the limb.

Lateral

This is a relative positional term referring to a place on the body being farther away from the midline than another point. For example, the ears are lateral to the eyes.

Levator scapula

This is a shoulder and neck muscle that attaches to the cervical vertebrae and the lateral base of the skull, elevating the scapulas. This muscle lies in the immediate vicinity of the upper trapezius and with it forms an area that is tight and sore on almost all adults.

Lomi lomi

Lomi lomi is a system of massage that utilizes very large, broad movements. Two-handed, forearm, and elbow application of strokes cover a broad area. Similar to Swedish massage in many aspects, this system uses prayer and the acknowledgment of the existence of a higher power as an integral part of the technique. Lomi lomi—Hawaiian for rub rub—is described by teacher Aunty Margaret Machado as "the loving touch—a connection between heart, hand, and soul with the source of all life."

Malleoli

This is a plural form of malleolis, or ankle bone. The medial malleolis is at the inferior end of the tibia, or larger lower leg bone, and the lateral malleolis is on the inferior end of the fibula, the smaller one. *Malleoli* is possibly the author's favorite English word, so it just had to be in the glossary. Also, it is a bony landmark that defines the space at the back of the heel below which is an important acupressure and reflexology point.

Mandible

This is a lower jaw bone. The bottom teeth are embedded in the mandible, and the mandible is part of the temperomandibular joint (TMJ) which is a hinge in front of the ear that allows for opening and closing the mouth.

Massage and massage therapy

These are systems of structured palpation and movement of the soft tissues of the body. The massage system may include such techniques as stroking, kneading, gliding, percussion, friction, vibration, compression, and passive or active stretching within the normal anatomical range of movement. The purpose of the practice of massage is to enhance the general health and well-being of the receiver.

Masseter

This is one of the two primary muscles which close the jaw, located between the zygomatic arch (the cheekbone) and the inferior edge of the lateral mandible.

Medial

This is a relative term that denotes a place on the body that is closer to the body's midline than another point. For example, the sacrum is medial to the hip.

Meridian Theory

This is the theory that meridians, or channels, make up a circuitry or giant web that delivers qi or life force energy to all of the organs and tissues of the body. This subtle energy system has been studied and treated in Traditional Chinese Medicine (TCM) for more than 5,000 years.

Occiput

This is the most posterior portion of the skull.

Occipital ridge

The most inferior portion of the occiput, where the back of the skull joins the top of the cervical spine (neck), is called the O.R.

Orbits

Orbits, or eye sockets, between the eyebrows at the base of the frontal bone of the skull, and the zygomatic arch (cheekbones).

Pain

Pain is any unpleasant sensation that can range from mild, localized discomfort to agony, with both physical and emotional components. Pain results from nerve stimulation, and may be isolated in an area or be more diffuse, as in disorders such as fibromyalgia.

Passive touch/contact hold

This is the practice of simply laying the fingers, one hand, or both hands on the receiver's body. Passive touch may impart heat to an area, have a calming influence, or help balance energy. Contact holds are an example of passive touch, and serve to introduce touch to the body at the beginning of a massage, when moving to a different area of the body, and for making a gentle exit at the end of a massage or when completing massage on one area of the body.

Parasympathetic nervous system response

This is a part of the nervous system response that serves to slow the heart rate, increase intestinal and gland activity, and allow for rest, relaxation, healing, and renewal in the body. These are opposite responses of the sympathetic nervous system (which accelerates the heart rate, constricts blood vessels, and raises blood pressure), which is the "fight or flight" part of the system. Almost all bodywork modalities seek to enhance the parasympathetic response and lower sympathetic nervous system excitation.

Pectoralis

These are the strong upper chest muscles that attach from the clavicle and sternum to the humerus (pectoralis major), and perform various movements of the upper arm and shoulder girdle. Pectoralis minor has attachments on the ribs and assists with movements of the shoulder girdle and raises the ribs for inhalation.

Petrissage

Petrissage is a Western massage technique category that includes movements that lift, wring, or squeeze soft tissues in a kneading motion; or press or roll the soft tissues under or between the hands.

Pinnae

This is the external part of the ear; made of cartilage.

Polarity therapy

This therapy is based on universal principles of energy: attraction, repulsion, and neutrality. The interrelation of these principles forms the basis for every aspect of life, including our experience of health, wellness, and disease. With this understanding, polarity therapy addresses the interdependence of body, mind, and spirit. Founded by Austrian-born naturopath Dr. Randolph Stone in the mid-1950s, polarity therapy is a clothes-on, noninvasive system complementing existing modalities with an integrated, holistic model.

Pronated
This is a position of the hands in which the palms are facing downward.

Prone
This is a position in which the entire body is lying face down.

Qi
Qi is the vital energy in a person, a construct of Asian bodywork. Qi is the energy that flows through the meridians of the body.

Quadriceps
These are the largest muscles of the thigh, which lie on the anterior, medial, and lateral sides of the thigh. They flex the hip and extend the knee, having an attachment immediately inferior to the patella, or kneecap.

Reflexology
This is a form of bodywork based on the theory of zone therapy, in which specific spots on the feet or hands are pressed to stimulate corresponding areas in other parts of the body. Reflexology is the practice of stimulating the hands and feet as a form of therapy. It has been observed that congestion or tension in any part of the foot mirrors congestion or tension in a corresponding part of the body.

Rocking
Rocking is the manipulation of a body part or parts with gentle or vigorous, rhythmic movements. It ends with the body part's return to its original position. Rocking reflexively relaxes tight muscles. Rocking is often used to treat joint problems, osteoarthritis, and tight muscles.

Sacrum
The Sacrum refers to the four or five fused vertebrae inferior to the lumbar spine; a hand-size bone that forms the posterior portion of the pelvis, and to which the ilia (bones of the ilium) attach laterally.

Scapula
The Scapula, or the shoulder blade, is located on the upper back, lateral to the vertebral column.

Shaking
Shaking is a movement performed by grasping either the muscle belly, for direct shaking, or the limb farthest away from the body, for indirect shaking. The tissue is then moved back and forth at an even rhythm—from gentle to vigorous. Shaking assists in increasing range of motion in a joint. It can be performed at the beginning, middle, or end of a massage and affects the sensory nerves in the muscles and joints, reducing muscle tightness.

Shiatsu
Shiatsu is a finger-pressure technique, developed in Japan, which utilizes traditional acupuncture points. Similar to acupressure, shiatsu concentrates on unblocking the flow of life energy and restoring balance in the meridians and organs to promote self-healing. With the receiver reclining, the giver applies pressure with the finger, thumb, palm, elbow, or knee to specific zones on the skin located along the energy meridians.

Spinous processes
This refers to the most posterior portions of the vertebrae. In the cervical region in particular, the spinous processes can be very delicate, and are subject to breakage if the bones have become weakened from osteoporosis.

Sternum
The sternum, or the breastbone, is a long, flat bone on the anterior chest, between the inferior neck and the abdomen.

Stripping
Stripping is a deep unidirectional stroke in which pressure is applied along muscle fibers with the fingertips, the ulnar border of the hand, the thumb, or the elbow.

Superior

This is a relational term referring to a place on the body that is farther upward than another place, as in the head is superior to the chest.

Supine

This refers to a position of the body as a whole, in which the person is lying face up.

Supinated

The position of the hands in which the palms are facing upward.

Swedish massage

A swedish massage is a vigorous system of treatment designed to energize the body by stimulating circulation. Five basic strokes, all flowing toward the heart, are used to manipulate the soft tissues of the body. Therapists use a combination of gliding, kneading, rolling, vibration, and percussive movements, with the application of lubricant to reduce friction on the skin. Swedish massage is one of the most commonly taught and well-known massage techniques.

Tantsu

Developed by Harold Dull, who also created Watsu, or water shiatsu, Tantsu (also known as Tantsu Tantric shiatsu) brings Watsu's in-water nurturing back onto land. In a Tantsu session, the giver cradles the receiver with her whole body. The receiver lies fully clothed on the floor, while the giver kneels or sits and supports the person. Like shiatsu, Tantsu is based on point work and powerful stretches to release chi (life force) along the body's meridians and in the energy centers, or chakras.

Tapotement

This is a Western massage therapy technique category consisting of brisk percussive movements that are performed in rapid rhythmic fashion. Forms of tapotement include hacking, cupping, slapping, tapping, and quacking.

Thai massage

Also called Nuad Bo-Rarn, Thai massage is body manipulation based on the theory that the body is made up of 72,000 sen, or energy lines, and applying pressure and stretch to these energy lines acts as an external stimulant to produce specific internal effects. Thai massage is practiced on a firm mat on the floor instead of on a table. Thai massage has been taught and practiced in Thailand for approximately 2,500 years.

Thrombosis

This is a thickening of blood from a liquid to a semisolid or solid structure that forms in the circulatory system's veins and arteries. Any indication or history of clots contraindicates massage which has the potential to loosen a thrombis, or clot, from the blood vessel wall, and allow it to move through the circulatory system and potentially to the brain, heart, or lungs, with serious health consequences.

Touch

To touch is to lay your hands upon something to come into contact with it. Massage therapists touch their clients or patients in many ways, but primarily with their hands. Touch may happen on a physical or an energetic level.

Traction

This is a slow, gentle pulling action with the body part along its axis, which causes the joint surface to slightly pull apart. Pulling or tractioning is performed in successive actions which nourishes the joint, helps to decrease muscle tone, and loosens any tissues that cross the joint being manipulated.

Trapezius

The Trapezius is a superficial back muscle with attachments on the vertebral column from the base of the skull to the lowest thoracic vertebra. The upper trapezius, which elevates the scapulas, is the area of the muscle that most frequently becomes tight and painful due to the activities of daily living and working and is one of the areas of the body on which most people appreciate massage.

Trochanter
See *Greater trochanter*.

Tubercle
See *Greater tubercle*.

Ventral
This is an area pertaining to the front of the body and frequently refers to the palms of the hands and soles of the feet.

Vertebral column
This is commonly called the spine orf back bone and consists of seven cervical (neck) vertebrae, twelve thoracic vertebrae each of which has ribs attached, and five lumbar vertebrae in the low back.

Vibration
This is a Western massage therapy technique category that includes oscillating, quivering, or trembling movements or movement of soft tissues back and forth or up and down, performed quickly and repeatedly. Vibration may be performed statically (in one place) or running (along the skin's surface).

Watsu
This is a form of aquatic shiatsu, which began at Harbin Hot Springs where Harold Dull brought his knowledge of Zen shiatsu into a warm pool. Zen shiatsu incorporates stretches that release blockages along the meridians—the channels through which chi or life force flows. Dull found the effects of Zen shiatsu could be amplified and made more profound by stretching someone while having her float in warm water.

Wellness massage
This is a massage performed with the intention of promoting the receiver's general well-being. It goes beyond the treatment of specific conditions to help the receiver achieve high-level wellness.

Wringing
Wringing is a type of rhythmic petrissage in which the whole hands are used to move muscle tissue back and forth between them in opposition, torquing the tissue and increasing mobility. Very similar in action to wringing water out of a towel.

Zen shiatsu
Zen shiatsu was developed by Shizuto Masanuga, who proposed the treatment of meridians beyond those recognized in the classical Chinese view. Masanuga also developed the widely accepted two-hand style, whereby one hand moves, applying pressure, while the other provides stationary support, and includes stretches along meridian lines.

Bibliography

Arledge, Garnette, and Jim, Harry Uhane. *Wise Secrets of Aloha: Learn and Live the Sacred Art of Lomilomi* (Weiser Books, 2007).

Avraham, Beatrice. *Thai Massage* (Astrolog Publishing House, 2001).

Beck, Mark F. *Milady's Theory and Practice of Therapeutic Massage*, Third Edition (Delmar Publishing, 1999).

Benjamin, Patricia J., and Tappan, Frances M. *Tappan's Handbook of Healing Massage Techniques: Classic, Holistic, and Emerging Methods*, Fourth Edition (Pearson Custom Publishing, 2005).

Bruder, Leslie. *Hot Stone Massage: A Three Dimensional Approach* (Lippincott, Williams and Wilkins, 2010).

Chai, Makana Risser Na Mo'olelo. *Lomilomi: The Traditions of Hawaiian Massage and Healing* (Bishop Museum Press, 2005).

Chow, Kam Thye. *Thai Yoga Massage: A Dynamic Therapy for Physical Wellbeing and Spiritual Energy* (Healing Arts Press, 2002).

Dougans, Inge, and Ellis, Suzanne. *Reflexology: Foot Massage for Total Health* (Barnes & Noble, 1991).

Dull, Harold. *Watsu: Freeing the Body in Water* (Trafford Press, 2004).

Dull, Harold, Ateeka, and Piane, Fabrizio Dalle. *Tantsu: A Yoga of the Heart* (Watsu Publishing, 2006).

Dull, Harold, and Piane, Fabrizio Dalle. "Core Tantsu" (video) (Watsu Publishing, 2007).

Gagh, Michael Reed. *Acupressure's Potent Points: A Guide to Self-care for Common Ailments* (Bantam Books, 1990).

Harris, Lynn. "The Sacred Heart of Hawaiian Lomi Lomi Massage" (video) (Lynn Harris Publications, 2008).

Hess, Mark, and Mochizuki, Shogo. *Japanese Hot Stone Massage* (Kotobiki Publications, 2002).

Lundberg, Paul. *The Book of Shiatsu* (Simon & Schuster, 2003).

Martin, Ingrid. *Aromatherapy for Massage Therapists* (Lippincott, Williams and Wilkins, 2007).

Masunaga, Shizuto, and Ohashi, Wataru. *Zen Shiatsu: How to Harmonize Yin and Yang for Better Health* (Japan Publications, Inc., 1977).

Rick, Stephanie. *The Reflexology Workout: Hand & Foot Massage for Super Health and Rejuvenation* (Harmony Books, 1986).

Salvo, Susan G. *Massage Therapy Principles and Practice* (Saunders Elsevier, 2007).

Somma, Corinna. *Shiatsu: A Complete Guide to Using Hand Pressure and Gentle Manipulation to Improve Your Health, Vitality, and Stamina* (Pearson—Prentice Hall, 2007).

Watson, Susan A., and Voner, Valerie. *Practical Reflexology: Interpretation and Techniques* (McGraw-Hill, 2009).

Resources

INFORMATION, ORGANIZATIONS, AND TRAINING

Western Massage and Bodywork Associations

Associated Bodyworkers & Massage Professionals (ABMP)
25188 Genesee Trail Road, Suite 200, Golden, CO, 80401
Phone: 800-458-2267
Fax: 800-667-8260
Email: expectmore@abmp.com
www.abmp.com

ABMP is an association of massage therapists and a clearinghouse for finding massage professionals in all bodywork specialties in the United States. It also offers information on massage therapy educational programs and continuing education.

American Massage Therapy Association (AMTA)
500 Davis Street, Suite 900, Evanston, IL, 60201-4695
Toll-free: 877-905-2700
Phone: 847-864-0123
Fax: 847-864-5196
Email: info@amtamassage.org
www.amtamassage.org

AMTA is an association of massage therapists and a clearinghouse for finding massage professionals in all bodywork specialties in the United States. It also offers information on massage therapy educational programs and continuing education.

American Polarity Therapy Association (APTA)
2888 Bluff Street, Suite 149, Boulder, CO, 803301
Tel: (303) 545-2080
Fax: (303) 545-2161
Website: www.polaritytherapy.org

Polarity therapy, a rapidly growing profession, comes under the guidance of the APTA, which registers and sets standards for the profession of polarity therapy. As a governing body, APTA has a code of ethics and an elected member board. It oversees educational standards, professional registration and ethics, national and international networking, and conferences.

Blue Ridge School of Massage and Yoga
2001 S. Main Street, Colony Park, Suite 106, Blacksburg, VA, 24060
Phone: 540-552-2177
Website: www.blueridgemassage.org

This school offers a 600-hour program in professional medical massage therapy, including Western and Eastern modalities.

Complementary Therapists Association (CThA)
PO Box 6955, Towcester, NN12 6WZ, United Kingdom
Phone: 0845 202 2941
Fax: 0844 779 8898
Email: info@complementary.assoc.org.uk

CThA is a leading organization representing more than 9,000 complementary therapists in the United Kingdom and Ireland.

Hawaiian Lomilomi Association

P.O. Box 2507, Kealakekua, HI, 96750-2356
Website: www.lomilomi.org

The Hawaiian Lomilomi Association (HLA) is an educational, nonprofit organization dedicated to organizing, promoting, and perpetuating the art of lomilomi, supporting Hawaiian culture and healing arts, and certifying the professional status of its members.

National Certification Board for Therapeutic Massage and Bodywork (NCBTMB)

1901 South Meyers Road, Suite 240, Oakbrook Terrace, IL 60181
Phone: 800-296-0664
Website: www.ncbtmb.org

NCBTMB is the certifying body for more than 90,000 NCBTMB-certified therapeutic massage therapists and bodyworkers in the United States. The organization provides information on certification, training programs, continuing education, and locating service for any kind of bodywork practitioner.

Reflexology Association of America

375 North Stephanie Street, Suite 1411, Henderson, NV, 89014
Administration Office:
PO Box 714, Chepachet, RI, 02814
Phone: 980-234-0159
Fax: 401-568-6449
Website: reflexology-usa.org

This is a nonprofit organization that promotes the scientific and professional advancement of reflexology. Its mission is to elevate and standardize the quality of reflexology services available to the public. It works to unify and support state reflexology associations to create one national movement toward greater excellence, integrity, research, and public safety.

Worldwide Aquatic Bodywork Association (WABA)

Harold Dull at P.O. Box 1817, Middletown, CA, 95461
Email: info@waba.edu
www.waba.edu

This association provides information on Tantsu and Watsu and other aquatic bodywork and shiatsu training. Look for Harold Dull's book, Tantsu® A Yoga of the Heart, and his DVDs. These as well as Tantsu classes can be found at www.tantsu.com.

Eastern or Asian Bodywork Associations

American Association of Acupuncture and Oriental Medicine (AAAOM)

PO Box 162340, Sacramento, CA, 95816
Toll Free: 866-455-7999
Phone: 916-443-4770
Fax: 916-443-4766
www.aaaomonline.org

One core purpose of AAAOM is to promote the professional field of acupuncture and Oriental medicine as a distinct, primary care field of medicine. AAAOM interacts with a wide range of organizations, institutions, and associations that oversee, govern, advance, or interact with the practice of acupuncture and Oriental medicine within the United States. AAAOM also offers information to educate the public regarding acupuncture and Oriental medicine.

American Organization for Bodywork Therapies of Asia (AOBTA)

1010 Haddonfield-Berlin Road, Suite 408, Voorhees, NJ, 08043-3514
Phone: 856-782-1616
Fax: 856-782-1653
Email: office@aobta.org

This is a nonprofit, professional membership organization representing instructors, practitioners, schools and programs, and students of Asian Bodywork Therapy (ABT).

International Thai Therapists Association (ITTA)

4715 Bruton Rd., Plant City, FL, 33565
Phone: 706-358-8646
Email: itta@core.com
Website: www.ThaiMassage.com
www.thaimassage.com/itta/ittaindex.html

This organization supports interest and accreditation in the yoga and therapeutic practice of Thai yoga, Thai massage, and traditional Thai-style bodywork and somatic practices.

Lotus Palm School and Certifying Thai Yoga Association

5244 Saint Urbain (near Fairmount), Montreal, Quebec, H2T 2W9, Canada
Phone: 514-270-5713
Fax: 514-270-8620
E-mail: info@lotuspalm.com
www.lotuspalm.com

This is Master teacher Kam Thye Chow's school and certifying organization for Thai Yoga Massage.

Shiatsu International Professional Associations

This is a professional body that regulates and publicizes shiatsu, with a clear code of ethics and conduct that ensure that their members have appropriate training to treat clients with respect and safety.

In Europe, two international bodies network among the countries and provide an interface with the European Union government. The European Shiatsu Federation (www.shiatsu-esf.org) represents the United Kingdom, Ireland, Spain, Belgium, The Czech Republic, Austria, Sweden, and Greece. The International Shiatsu Network (www.shiatsunetwork.com) represents Germany, France, and Switzerland.

In Italy, however, six organizations represent shiatsu. Go to www.shiatsuinfo.org/associations.shtml for more information on them, including the largest, Federazione Italiana Shiatsu (FIS).

In the United States, shiatsu is regulated by the American Organization for Bodywork Therapies of Asia (www.aobta.org); in Canada, by the Shiatsu Society of Canada (www.shiatsupractor.org); and in Australia, by the Shiatsu Therapy Association of Australia (www.staa.org.au).

MASSAGE MATERIALS AND SUPPLIES

Bodyworkmall

200 E. South Temple, Suite 190
Salt Lake City, UT 84111
Phone: 866-717-6753
Fax: 801-363-2038
www.bodyworkmall.com

Massage Warehouse & Spa Essentials

This company carries everything for massage, from tables to lubricants, mats, stones, and more.
Phone: 800-910-9955
www.massagewarehouse.com

Earthlite Massage Tables and Supplies

800-872-0560
www.earthlite.com

This is a supplier of a wide range of eco-friendly and well-designed and sturdy professional massage tables, tables for home use, and associated massage equipment and products.

Rub Rocks

5071 David Strickland Road #103, Fort Worth, TX, 76119
Phone: 800-941-0231
http://rubrocks.com
Email: webhelp@rubrocks.com
www.rubrocks.com

This is a supplier of hot and cold stones for massage; the best source for a wide variety of stones and equipment for hot stone massage

Acknowledgments

Thanks for the patience, support, and encouragement of my beloved friends who have remained in touch even when I've been preoccupied; to my fellow instructors at Blue Ridge School of Massage and Yoga, who took on additional responsibilities while I have been writing; to all those students of massage over the past thirteen years who have taught me how to communicate the essentials of massage practice; and to all the wonderful massage therapy clients, who've given me abundant opportunities to practice my craft.

For content, I would like to thank Jeff Tiebout, my business partner and original massage instructor, for the grounding in massage basics and in Swedish massage and an introduction to shiatsu. I bow to Elisha Reygle's knowledge of reflexology; to Lynn Harris's artful instruction in lomi lomi; to Harold Dull for his creative genius in developing and teaching Watsu and Tantsu; to Minakshi for her instruction in meridian theory and Watsu; to Kam Thye Chow for his graceful transmission of Thai yoga massage; and to all the authors and presenters who have given so generously of their knowledge and creativity in the ever-broadening field of bodywork.

Special thanks to Earthlite for providing the massage table for the photos in this book and to Rub Rocks for providing a set of stones for the photos of hot stone massage.

In Gratitude,

Victoria Jordan Stone, CMT

About the Author

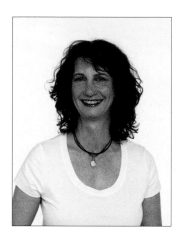

Victoria Jordan Stone, nationally certified massage therapist, began massage training to supplement her hospice volunteer work in 1989, not expecting massage therapy to become an occupation. Receiving massage therapy had proved vital in restoring her health and well-being following a serious back injury in 1987 and also helped to reduce the stress of operating an ad agency. She found she wanted to help others with their discomforts as she had been helped.

She has specialized in various forms of clinical massage including deep tissue massage; trigger-point therapies; massage in pregnancy; Swedish, myofascial release, cranio-sacral therapy, movement, and hot stone massage; Watsu aquatic bodywork; Thai yoga massage; and reiki, polarity, and lomi lomi massage. She is a Yoga Alliance-registered yoga instructor and a birth doula.

She has also taught couples massage since 1992 and professional massage therapy classes since 1996, becoming a partner in the Blue Ridge School of Massage and Yoga in 2000, where she continues as academic director and one of the primary instructors at the school in Blacksburg, Virginia. In April 2007, her book, *The Complete Idiot's Guide to Massage Illustrated*, was published by Penguin Press. One of the models for the book, photographed by Bob Shell, is Victoria's daughter Sasha, also a massage therapist.

Index